Responding to the AIDS Challenge

A comparative study of local AIDS programmes in the United Kingdom

Edited by
Maryan Pye, Mukesh Kapila,
Graham Buckley and Deirdre Cunningham

Responding to the AIDS Challenge

A comparative study of local AIDS programmes in the United Kingdom

Edited by
Maryan Pye, Mukesh Kapila,
Graham Buckley and Deirdre Cunningham

Longman Group UK Limited
Industry and Public Service Management Division
Westgate House, The High,
Harlow, Essex, CM20 1YR

First published 1989

A CIP catalogue record   this book is available
from The British Library

ISBN 0582 064341

Design by Philip Mann /ACE Ltd
Typeset by DP Photosetting, Aylesbury, Bucks
Printed and bound in Great Britain by
Biddles Ltd, Guildford, Surrey

Contents

The Contributors

Dr Peter Anderson   General practitioner and Senior Registrar in Community Medicine. Has been involved in research into the management of HIV in general practice.

Virginia Blakey   Head of Special Programmes at Health Promotion Authority for Wales since July 1988. Responsible for the Authority's AIDS programme.

Dr Graham Buckley   General practitioner, Livingston, West Lothian. Chairman of HIV and AIDS Working Party of the Royal College of General Practitioners.

Mr S. Cavicchia   Health education officer to the Sussex AIDS Centre and Helpline since June 1987, with a background in voluntary work in the drugs and HIV field.

Dr Deirdre Cunningham   Director of Public Health, Parkside Health Authority, and Medical Officer for Environmental Health, City of Westminster, London. Member of the National Association of Health Authorities Working Party on AIDS, and the AIDS Services Working Group (Department of Health). Chair of the Faculty of Community Medicine Working Party on AIDS.

Dr Philip A. Gaskell   Principal in General Practice in north central Edinburgh, experienced in caring for people with HIV infection and promoting support and education for colleagues in general practice.

Dr Rob George   Senior Lecturer in Palliative and Community Care. Academic Department of Genito-urinary Medicine, University College and Middlesex School of Medicine; Physician, Honorary Consultant, Middlesex Hospital; Consultant Physician on a multidisciplinary community-based team providing terminal and community care for people with HIV-related disease.

Dr Graham Hart   Lecturer in Medical Sociology, Academic Department of Genito-urinary Medicine, University College and Middlesex School of Medicine; Research interests include the health beliefs and health behaviour of gay men in relation to HIV and AIDS.

Christopher J. Hayes   District Health Promotion Officer, North West Hertfordshire Health Authority. Responsible for leading the district's HIV/AIDS team and preparation of the district strategy.

Dr A. Iversen   Specialist in Community Medicine, Brighton Health Authority, lead officer in the authority for HIV infection and AIDS issues.

Dr Mukesh Kapila   Specialist in Community Medicine and Deputy Director of the AIDS Programme, Health Education Authority and Temporary Adviser to the World Health Organization Global Programme on AIDS.

Dr M. Paula J. Kilbane Specialist in Community Medicine, Eastern Health and Social Services Board. Chairman of the AIDS Steering Group. Member of the Faculty of Community Medicine AIDS Working Group.

Mr Gorm D. Kirsch HIV prevention and care facilitator, Oxfordshire Health Authority, involved in developing primary health care responses. Has previously worked with HIV/AIDS in voluntary agencies and statutory bodies in the US and UK.

Dr Gordon R. Macphail Until recently, a general practitioner in Brighton with considerable experience in caring for people with HIV infection and AIDS. Currently working in the field of palliative care for people with AIDS.

Dr Agnes McKnight Senior Lecturer, Department of General Practitioners, Queen's University Belfast; member of the AIDS Steering Group, Eastern Health and Social Services Board.

Dr Kathie Marfell Specialist in Community Medicine, Bradford Health Authority; Medical Officer for Environmental Health, Bradford Metropolitan District Council; AIDS Co-ordinator and Chair of Bradford Health Authority standing HIV Action Group.

Dick Mayon-White Specialist in Community Medicine (Epidemiology) and consultant responsible for the control of communicable disease; Chairman of AIDS Taskforce, Oxfordshire Health Authority. Has undertaken studies of general practitioners' and public's knowledge of AIDS.

Ms Fiona O'Donnell AIDS/HIV education co-ordinator, responsible for co-ordinating the AIDS Awareness Programme; member of the Central Training Team and school writing group for the Eastern Health and Social Services Board in Northern Ireland.

Richard Parish Chief of Operations Division at the Health Promotion Authority for Wales.

Dr Maryan Pye Special Adviser to the Health Education Authority's AIDS programme. Formerly a district-based specialist in Community Medicine with responsibilities for health promotion and co-ordinating the local response to HIV and AIDS.

Debbi Reid Formerly education and training officer with the Welsh AIDS Campaign. Now health promotion adviser on AIDS at the Health Promotion Authority for Wales.

Dr Alison M. Richardson Principal Clinical Psychologist for HIV and AIDS, Lothian Health Board. Honorary Fellow, Edinburgh University.

Paul Roderick MA, MRCP Registrar in Community Medicine, Parkside Health Authority. Has been involved in developing the district's AIDS strategy, a minimum data set on HIV/AIDS, the evaluation of a needle exchange scheme and the development of a strategy for drug users and HIV.

Andrew Stevens MB, BS, MSc
Senior Registrar in Community
Medicine, Parkside Health Authority.
Has been involved in developing the
district's AIDS strategy and is a member
of the Faculty of Community Medicine
AIDS Working Group.

Mrs June C. Whitham   AIDS co-
ordinator, City of Bradford
Metropolitan Council, responsible for
the overall direction and control of the
AIDS prevention strategy and the
management of initiatives such as the
needle exchange scheme.

Dr Peter Willis   General practitioner
and Clinical Assistant in Genito-urinary
Medicine; general practitioner
representative on Bloomsbury AIDS
Steering Group and has experience of
HIV and AIDS in primary care.

Dr Anne Wright   District Medical
Officer, North West Hertforshire
Health Authority. Chair, District AIDS
Action Group, and member, North
West Thames Regional HIV Planning
Group. Member of Faculty of
Community Medicine AIDS Working
Group since 1984.

Preamble and Preliminaries

Dr Maryan Pye

Calamity of every kind – war, famine, pestilence, catastrophe, injustice, oppression and natural disaster – is, historically speaking, routine in human experience, much as we in the rich nations of the so-called first world would like to pretend otherwise. And routinely we respond, conservatively, piecemeal and often very late in the day. We congratulate ourselves for not throwing money at problems. We investigate, report, recommend, legislate, raise standards, develop technologies, reorganise and restructure. But often we continue substantially as before, until calamity takes us by surprise once more.

Yet history also shows that, from time to time, the human race is confronted by crises which impact in a quite different, profound and transforming way, the repercussions sounding across every boundary and population as well as on the pattern of life for future generations. These are the events which bring both unimaginable crisis and great challenge; events that expose the fabric of society where it is worn out or rotten through and through and, in doing so, stir the human spirit out of its habitual complacency to insist on, and fight for, a reponse that is focused on fundamental and far-reaching change. I believe, that in our time, AIDS is such an event and that history will judge this generation by the quality of our response.

Christopher Spence
Director, London Lighthouse

The appearance of the epidemic of HIV infection and AIDS in the 1980s poses a great challenge to the promotion and preservation of public health in the United Kingdom. Part of the crisis is the enormous burden of care for those whose lives have been disrupted by the infection, whose needs are special and whose carers have often been confused and uncertain. At the same time, in the absence of technological means to cure or prevent, we are called upon to mount a preventive exercise for the whole population, which, at an individual level, might be regarded as intrusive, impractical or even offensive.

An analysis of the problems confronted by those working in the field of HIV infection and AIDS reveals that few of the details are new. We have in the past confronted infections which are transmitted by sexual or blood-to-blood contact and for which there is no cure. We have identified the problems of confidentiality, of care in the community, of facing up to life-threatening diseases and of dying with dignity and in peace. Health educators have had to address issues of sexuality relating to disease transmission and to unplanned pregnancies and as part of the curriculum of personal and social education. In addition, there is, sadly, nothing new about prejudice towards those whose sexual orientation or lifestyle, by choice or otherwise, is beyond the comprehension of the majority.

What is new is that these issues arise together, focused on the effects of a particular virus, at this point in our social history. There has been an enormous range of responses to a multiplicity of problems. On a national scale, the government has allocated funding for caring services and preventive action and has initiated an educational campaign which has already had major influences on our society. Topics once discussed in hushed tones, behind closed doors or accompanied by sniggers, are nowadays the subject of general conversation. Awareness of HIV and AIDS has also revealed areas of weakness in the way in which health and social services operate – for example, the lack of staff training programmes and inadequate arrangements for the disposal of clinical waste.

The multiplicity of responses to the challenge of AIDS reflects the creative thinking and innovative ways of working which have been directed to this problem; but it also demonstrates the hurdles, which have to be surmounted in order to provide effective services. This book examines some of the ways in which different parts of the country have tackled the problem of HIV infection. A range of solutions – some more successful than others – are described with a view to sharing experiences with those who confront similar issues. An attempt is also made to view the responses to AIDS in the context of a model of public health.

Background to the project

The Health Education Authority (HEA), the Royal College of General Practitioners (RCGP) and the Faculty of Community Medicine (FCM) share, along with many others, a commitment to the prevention of the spread of HIV infection with minimal harmful social disruption. In the spring of 1988, representatives of these three organisations met together, and an idea was generated to 'review and document the experiences of those working in selected parts of the United Kingdom in order to bring together common themes, key experiences, examples of successful approaches and lessons that may be recommended to others'. To this end, it was decided to invite a range of 'case-study' reports outlining the local responses to AIDS in a number of different locations.

A small steering group was formed, the membership of which has been ultimately responsible for the editing of this book. The Health Education Authority's AIDS programme was responsible for financial support and commissioned a project worker to oversee the production, collation, editing and analysis and to comment on the various contributions.

Selection of contributors

The selection of locations and contributors was neither random nor was it highly selective. The aim was to find a mix of areas with high and low prevalence of HIV infection. The intention was to examine and contrast the response to what may have first presented as a hospital-based problem with a major clinical workload with an essentially preventive approach for which the chief problem may be maintaining momentum. At the same time, we wanted to include not just London but other major cities, and to compare them with more rural population centres and the commuter areas in between. Locations were selected to represent different population mixes – of age structure, ethnic background, levels of employment, social class, politics and culture. Inclusion of all parts of the United Kingdom ensured a wide geographical spread and a variety of organisational responses.

We wanted to illustrate the wide range of HIV preventive work that we felt sure was happening; we did not invite contributions because we thought they would be the 'best' or even the 'worst' examples. In most cases, initial links in each area were made through contact with general practitioners and community physicians. Not all the people we asked had the time or the resources to contribute, but eventually nine locations agreed to participate in the project by each producing a local report and commentary on the reports of others. Local knowledge produced a team of two or three contributors from each patch, and serendipity contributed to the formation of a multi-disciplinary, multi-agency, industrious and enthusiastic writing team.

How we worked together

The group met together twice. The first workshop in London in June 1988 allowed us to get to know one another and to find out the past and current range of activities in each district and the particular interests of the contributors. At that time, a lengthy checklist of requirements for each section was drawn up and agreed. During the summer, the writing teams worked at producing their first drafts.

As part of my co-ordinating role, I was able to visit nearly all the writers to discuss the local issues which seemed most important, and to learn much more about the local programmes for HIV and AIDS prevention, including some of the less overt difficulties encountered. It became clear that to capture the total content of nine local AIDS programmes would have been an impossible task. The concluding section of this book draws on some of the local and group discussions on topics not necessarily mentioned elsewhere in the text.

By September 1988, the first drafts were completed and circulated among other members of the group for comment. A second workshop was convened in Manchester in October 1988. For an intensive 24 hours, a peer-group appraisal and case-study analysis took place. Initially, each individual case study was scrutinised by the group both in relation to its content and to its style. Some individuals expressed real interest in what others (particularly the authors) considered mundane. The wealth of background detail for each location, although of interest at an individual level, was felt to contribute little to the overall content. After rethinking the style of the reports, participants agreed to rewrite their contributions, this time not as a series of comprehensive local reports, but as more detailed illustrations of themes suggested by the group. Members of the steering group and the participants then worked through an analysis of all the case studies, drawing out common themes and contrasting responses and relating them to their particular local situations.

The rest of the story is simply that of the editorial process, which entailed each writing team agreeing not only their own contribution but also taking responsibility for at least one other. At the end of the day, although this is essentially a collection of writings, it is also very much the product of a group effort, both in its formulation and analysis.

The contents

The aim of the Health Education Authority's AIDS programme is concerned with the prevention of HIV transmission without harmful social impact. As part of this process, the HEA is committed to the development and advocacy of effective health promotion policies and the dissemination of examples of good practice. The concerns of the Faculty of Community Medicine and the Royal College of General Practitioners also encompass the nature and quality of services provided for those with HIV infection and AIDS.

In practice, preventing the spread of HIV infection cannot be seen in isolation from the care of those already infected: indeed, spread of infection may be as dependent on the behaviour of those who are infectd as it is on those who are not. In addition, in the caring situation, appropriate training and support for carers will improve their confidence and, with it, the quality and safety of the care that they provide.

Thus the topics addressed here reflect the range of activities undertaken by the members of the writing teams, either where HIV/AIDS is the main focus of their work or where it impacts on their day-to-day work in related fields. Of the 23 local contributors, 7 are community physicians, 8 are working in the broad field of health education and 8 are practitioners working with individuals in clinical situations; 5 of these practitioners are in general practice.

High-prevalence districts

Some of the districts were identified as those where the initial response to HIV and AIDS arose from the need to provide services for people with AIDS. Historically, the London districts were the first to be confronted by this situation. From **Paddington and North Kensington**, we learn how the organisational response has developed over time, with a shifting power base for decision-making and resource allocation. This has moved from a clinical base with research funding to a management base with health authority funding. There is also a glimpse of some local issues such as housing and prostitution. The response to caring for people outside hospital is described through the development of the Support Team, and the voluntary sector initiative in building the London Lighthouse, a residential care facility for people with HIV and AIDS.

In **Bloomsbury**, there has been a parallel organisational response. This case study goes on to explore in depth the response to two particular inner city problems: services for drug users, including primary care and health promotion; and the co-ordination and support required for care in the community for people with AIDS who do not wish or need to be in hospital.

Drug problems are also central to the report from **Lothian** where there is a high prevalence of HIV infection among injecting drug users. Here, current problems are exacerbated by a lack of appropriate provision in the past, but new initiatives are under way. From Edinburgh, we learn of the impact of this new type of caseload for general practitioners, one for which they may feel ill equipped (or possibly disinclined) to cope. This rather negative view is balanced by the tremendous contribution made by some general practitioners in providing care and in educating colleagues about drug problems and HIV infection.

A view from general practice is provided by a practitioner whose work spans these two London districts. He describes at a personal level some of the problems faced by caring for people with HIV and AIDS.

Moving to the less urban situation in **Brighton**, we have a different model of organisational change in response to HIV/AIDS and an illustration of the valuable role played by the voluntary sector, which has evolved to become a broad-based organisation working in concert with the statutory sector. A former general practitioner with local experience highlights some of the difficulties experienced in providing appropriate primary care in the community for people with AIDS and HIV disease.

Low-prevalence districts

Co-operation between health and local authorities in **Oxford** at an early stage resulted in the innovative joint appointment of an AIDS Liaison Officer. Experience gained from this post is described, along with an examination of other organisational responses, including relationships with the university. There is local experience of 'facilitators' working with general practitioners in health promotion, specifically in the prevention of heart disease. This model has been used, apparently with success, to support general practitioners in preparing to care for the effects, and to prevent the spread, of HIV infection. Oxford is also the regional centre for haemophilia and the comments on the 'separateness' of these patients may be familiar to those working in other such regional centres.

In **Bradford**, the impending epidemic of HIV and AIDS is viewed as a potential public health problem. The collaborative response of the health and local authorities is described, including preventive initiatives ranging from needle exchange to media promotions. The population of Bradford includes a significant number from ethnic minority groups, for whom English is neither their first language nor their usual culture. This report emphasises the importance of the cultural context, and AIDS health promotion is proposed as part of a broad initiative in the promotion of health.

From **North West Hertfordshire**, an affluent commuter area, we learn of the way in which a pro-active reponse has been mounted for health education and with the voluntary sector. In a detailed study, the sexual experiences and educational needs of another special audience – people with mental handicap – are described.

From the Eastern Health and social services Board in **Belfast**, there is another example of setting up education and staff training programmes in advance of the pressures of clinical problems. An education programme for schools has been established which takes account of the particular cultural sensitivities of Northern Ireland. This has, in turn, provided considerable support for a previously identified need for general programmes of sex education. Once more, the educational and anticipated support needs of general practitioners are considered, and a slightly different model is proposed for the role of a 'general practitioner facilitator' working in general practice.

From **Wales**, the case study is confined to a consideration of health promotion. The Health Promotion Authority for Wales has responsibilities which are similar to those of the Health Education Authority in England, but on a scale more comparable to a large English health region. Although progress has been hindered by organisational change and the associated disruption and uncertainty, a wide range of programme activities and basic research has been implemented.

This is essentially a collection of highly individual writings, guided by the group as a whole. It is not intended to be a comprehensive listing of the contents of local AIDS programmes, neither does it purport to describe the right or the best approach to some of the difficulties with which those working in the field of HIV and AIDS are becoming familiar. We hope to provide an opportunity to share experiences, to learn, to adapt and to feed back. Networks are becoming firmly established, not only through bodies such as the Health Education Authority, the Faculty of Community Medicine and the Royal College of General Practitioners but also through local and national links between health and local authorities and the voluntary sector.

It is our intention that this book should be read by a diverse audience which might include public health physicians, general practitioner, AIDS workers, health promoters, planners, managers, politicians, teachers – indeed, everyone who has an interest in preventing the spread of HIV infection. It will have succeeded in its aim if it provokes comment and discussion, and sows the seeds for new initiatives in health promotion relating to HIV and AIDS.

Note from the editors: The case study reports reflect the personal views of the authors, often following extensive local discussion. They have not been formally agreed by the relevant health authorities and should not be taken as statements of official policy.

Fighting the Fire in Paddington and North Kensington

Paul Roderick and Andrew Stevens

With 126,000 people living in four square miles of inner London, Paddington and North Kensington (PNK) was the smallest and most densely populated health district in Britain. Even so, the number of permanent residents declined continuously over the last century, reaching its nadir in 1983. Following the merger with Brent in April 1988, PNK now forms part of Parkside Health District.

The social make-up of the area could hardly be more varied, ranging from the leafy townhouse area of Holland Park to the highly deprived area adjacent to the Westway flyover. Despite the presence of wealthy areas, the district rates as the second worst on the Department of Environment's deprivation index (Department of Environment, 1983). There is a large

Figure 1 **Paddington and North Kensington Health Authority**

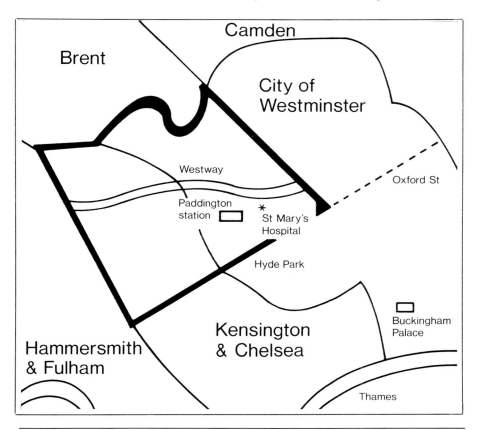

ethnic minority population, with 16.5 per cent of heads of households born in the New Commonwealth or Pakistan. A very large number of temporarily homeless people from all over London are accommodated in a tight cluster of bed-and-breakfast hotels near Paddington Station. The local population is highly mobile, with an approximately 30 per cent turnover every year; and there is a higher proportion of young adults than in the population of the UK as a whole.

The district's main hospital, St Mary's, is one of the principal London teaching hospitals and is located right next to Paddington Station. Of the district's 81 general practitioners, 55 per cent are single-handed and often elderly GPs who work in adverse conditions. Demand for open-access hospital services is therefore high, stemming from the problems of inner city deprivation and day-time commuters, as well as from the balance between primary and hospital care facilities.

A particular sphere of the hospital's activity, which is out of all proportion to the size of the local population, is the use made of the Genito-urinary Medicine (GUM) Clinic (Praed Street Clinic). This applies as much, if not more, to people with AIDS or HIV infection as to people presenting with other sexually transmitted diseases. PNK was the second largest reporting district for AIDS in the UK, although only a quarter of the total number were resident in the district. Table 1 shows the number of people with AIDS diagnosed in the district from June 1983 (the first St Mary's case) to December 1988, when a total of 326 cases had been diagnosed. Of these, at least 174 are known to have died.

Table 1 **Numbers of people with AIDS diagnosed and reported from PNK 1984–8**

	Diagnosed/treated	*Known to have died*
Pre-1984	12	3
1984	32	10
1985	34	23
1986	77	44
1987	81	42
1988	90	52
Total	326	174

The pressures created by the HIV epidemic were being met in a resource-losing district. With a large teaching hospital and a declining population, PNK has inevitably been subject to financial stringency. A series of district budget deficits and crisis-laden health authority meetings have coincided exactly with the increasing demands created by the HIV epidemic. Inevitably this background has played a part in how the district has responded to the HIV phenomenon (Ferlie and Pettigrew, 1988).

The breadth of the response

Notwithstanding the financial difficulties that the district faced during the early and mid-1980s, the response to HIV has been far reaching. By mid-1988, the district had, in the acute services, designated a specific AIDS ward, commenced the expansion of the Praed Street Clinic and established a follow-up clinic (the Wharfside Clinic) and Home Support Team for patients after discharge. Voluntary testing services with pre- and post-test counselling are provided at the Praed Street Clinic and the Drug Dependency Unit (DDU). Health promotion – with an emphasis on avoiding risky behaviour – is promulgated to identified groups and, where appropriate, to the general population. A specific preventive measure has been the establishment of a needle exchange scheme. Also within the district are some other facilities of note:

- The North West Thames Regional HIV Health Education Project (managed by the district) which provides health education resources for districts and researchers on specific HIV health education topics.
- The London Lighthouse, a charitable foundation providing an alternative to hospital care.
- The National AIDS Counselling Unit which developed from local experience gained by the district's clinical psychologists and health advisers. This is a training facility open to anyone involved in HIV-related work.

The local authorities overlapping the district's boundaries – Westminster and Kensington & Chelsea – have also been concerned with AIDS awareness and services.

This range of facilities says little about their relative importance or of the machinations required to establish them. To a great extent, the district response has been dominated by the acute services. The history of these services has been very chequered and has been mirrored only by the other two (adjacent) districts in the country that also have sizeable numbers of AIDS cases: Bloomsbury and Riverside. Other developments in the district have not been greatly different from those elsewhere, but there are some aspects that have been interesting or unique. In particular, these include: the development of the Home Support Team; the response to housing needs of

AIDS patients; the development of the London Lighthouse; and the relevance of female prostitution to the HIV epidemic.

The history of the acute services' response

St Mary's Hospital developed as one of the three major centres in the United Kingdom for the diagnosis and treatment of HIV infection and AIDS. This can be ascribed to two main factors.

First, there has always been a strong tradition of virology and microbiology at St Mary's. When the first reports came from the United States about the appearance of opportunistic infections and Kaposi's sarcoma developing in homosexuals, three consultants (including two from these disciplines) anticipated that this problem would develop in the United Kingdom. At the same time, a clinical immunologist with a strong research and clinical interest in the infectious complications of immuno-suppressive disorders was appointed to St Mary's. In 1982, these four consultants commenced the first cohort study of homosexual patients in the United Kingdom (funded by the Wellcome Trust).

Second, the Praed Street Clinic, Europe's largest open access GUM clinic, has always served a large gay population, and it has maintained a sympathetic attitude to this group of patients.

The dramatic adaptation of St Mary's to the AIDS epidemic is summarised in Figure 2, which shows the numbers of cases, the money allocated and the main decision-making areas. As can be seen, the specific AIDS finance made available from the DHSS via the regional health authority lagged behind the caseload. The changing decision-making structure can be interpreted to some extent as a response to the money available.

A great range of events contributed to the AIDS response, and these are summarised in Table 2, which gives the chronology of the main events both nationally and locally. The development of HIV and AIDS services within the district can be considered in four overlapping phases.

1982–4: Beginnings – the District Control of Infection Committee phase

With the homosexual cohort study and the keen interest of the four consultants, St Mary's attracted, through the media and among the gay copmmunity, a national reputation in the research field. The first patients with AIDS provoked an acute crisis among hospital staff, and medical staff had to undertake frontline efforts to educate staff groups about HIV infection. The situation was made more difficult by recurrent sensational media reports. Following this staff education and the development of infection control policies by the District's Control of Infection Committee (DCIC), people with AIDS were treated in the hospital in increasing numbers. There was a reluctance by other clinicians to be involved at this stage, and so it fell primarily on the clinical immunologist and the genito-urinary physician to treat all people with, respectively, AIDS and HIV infection. The DCIC played a role in bed allocations, which were designated on the infectious disease ward.

Figure 2 AIDS cases, funds and decision-making areas 1982–9

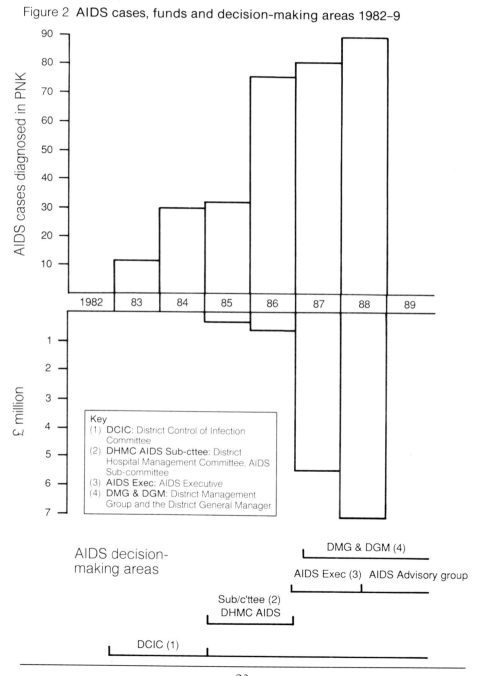

The key consultants of the three major centres for AIDS in London – St Mary's, St Stephen's and the Middlesex – achieved national media prominence as unofficial spokesmen on AIDS, and they lobbied the Department of Health and Social Security to take a lead in developing a national strategy and to provide funding. Faced with difficulties in their dealings with their general practitioners and local communities, gay men tended to turn more to the acute hospitals for care and support. Experience in counselling people with HIV and AIDS developed because of the specific interest of one health adviser and two clinical psychologists.

Funding of AIDS care at this stage was not a major issue as the numbers were relatively small, and some money did come from research grants. The first specific funding bid, related to acute care, was initiated for 1985/6 by the clinical immunologist.

1983–6: The District Hospital Medical Committee phase

As the number of patients with HIV and AIDS attending the hospital increased, and despite the fact that it had become clearer that an American-style HIV epidemic would develop in the UK, resistance to the development of AIDS services grew among some clinicians not directly involved. Nevertheless, specific DHSS funding became available for AIDS, and the District Hospital Medical Committee (DHMC) took over from the District Control of Infection Committee with the prime aim of steering bids for this money. These bids were led largely by clinicians and pathologists with very little emphasis on community care or health education. General management had, by this time, been introduced to the district, but at this stage it played a largely reactive role.

A major development in September 1985 was the introduction of HIV testing of all blood donations and the resulting need for alternative open-access testing sites. The Praed Street Clinic became one such site and was faced with an increasing number of people requesting testing. The health advisers, who are contact tracers and counsellors in the GUM clinic, anticipated this need by producing a leaflet describing the test and offering pre- and post-test counselling.

Counselling in the district developed apace with the interest of the clinical psychology department. At first, everyone was counselled by a psychologist, but the increase in numbers soon necessitated a two-tier system with health advisers doing the initial counselling and referring on those needing further help. The DHSS recognised this local expertise by basing the National AIDS Counselling Unit at St Mary's Hospital in 1985.

In-patients with AIDS were mostly managed on the 12-bed infectious disease ward, and clinicians became concerned about the expansion of bed usage by patients with AIDS as well as staff involvement with them, particularly in the intensive care unit. Some surgeons were antagonistic and wanted to wear 'spacesuits' and screen all patients for HIV antibodies. The

Table 2 A national and local chronology of the response to AIDS

Medium	The national epidemic	The government response	The regional and district response	Local authorities and the voluntary sector
1981	First UK AIDS case.			
1982			Homosexual cohort study.	
1983	'Gay plague' media message.	High-risk groups asked not to give blood.	First St Mary's AIDS case.	
1984				First Terrence Higgins Trust Helpline.
1985		DHSS expert advisory group set up. Blood donor and alternative site testing.	Regional AIDS Working Party. District Control of Infection policy issued. AIDS beds set at 8. National AIDS Counselling Unit set up at St Mary's.	
1986		DHSS requires district AIDS plans. £20 million publicity campaign.	Two-tier counselling system with health advisers and psychologists.	
1987	1,000 AIDS cases reported.	DHSS Community Care conference. AIDS (Control) Act. AZT available. Health Education Authority given AIDS brief.	Home Support Team. Needle-exchange scheme. Staff employment policy (on confidentiality). 200th district case.	Start of health authority and local authority joint AIDS planning.
1988			AIDS beds doubled. Opening of follow-up clinic.	Local authorities get direct AIDS funding. London Lighthouse opens.

DHMC tried to restrict to eight the number of in-patients with AIDS, but this was not acceptable to the consultants responsible for AIDS care. It was, however, agreed that there should be no more referrals from other hospitals and that patients should be referred back to their district of residence wherever possible. However, they were reluctant to be treated in their own districts as HIV/AIDS services at that time were rudimentary other than in the three main 'AIDS districts' in London. A major problem was the absence of adequate surveillance and monitoring of case numbers. This meant that attempts at managerial control had to take place in a climate more of hype than rationality. This deficit was rectified in the next phase.

1986–8: The AIDS Executive phase
From late 1986, there were some signs of a shift away from the predominantly hospital-based approach to one which at least considered community care. The District General Manager felt that too much emphasis had been put on acute care and that the bids for money were excessive and sometimes inappropriate. The increasing number of people with AIDS treated as in-patients was putting extra pressure on a declining number of acute beds. A new District Medical Officer (DMO) then arrived who was keen to be involved in developing a comprehensive strategy for AIDS and HIV which would include the development of community and terminal care, health education and better links with local authorities, as well as pushing for proper surveillance of the numbers of people in the district with diagnosed AIDS and HIV infection.

A new body was formed called the AIDS Executive, exclusively health authority staffed and chaired by the DMO. A wider group – of which the AIDS Executive was the core, and including the local authorities and voluntary organisations – was also formed, but it did not make serious collaborative progress and met only once, deciding that the existing joint planning mechanisms were a more appropriate means of liaison. These existed within each of the two local authorities, and so it was agreed that the two be merged for AIDS purposes. However, disagreements between the two local authorities meant that this body too met only once and liaison proceeded separately thereafter.

The AIDS Executive, meanwhile, set out to develop a strategy and an operational plan to develop services using the increasing allocation of funds earmarked for AIDS by the DHSS. A District Planner was co-opted on to the group to help with this process. The main principles of the AIDS strategy, produced in early 1988 and mainly written by the DMO and her staff, are set out in the box below. The AIDS Executive agreed the principle that AIDS is essentially the same as any other major disease. As such, services should be drawn into and from existing systems, without the need for superimposed or *ad hoc* committees (often without executive authority).

Paddington and North Kensington AIDS Strategy (1988): Summary of Aims

The district's AIDS strategy was produced in the first quarter of 1988 in order to plan district-based services for HIV and to give a co-ordinated direction to the various services which had already developed. There are particular problems faced in developing such a strategy:

- The size of the epidemic: there are now over 1,500 cases in the UK and an estimated 50,000–100,000 HIV-positive individuals.
- Its concentration in three Inner London health authorities (Riverside, Parkside, Bloomsbury).
- The complex and expensive therapy used to control its clinical manifestation in the absence of a cure or vaccine.
- Public attitudes and stigmatisation which necessitate maximum confidentiality and prevent easy dissemination of information.

The main aims of the strategy are:

1. To prevent the spread of HIV infection by increasing people's understanding of the disease, its methods of transmission and ways of avoiding exposure to the virus.
2. To develop appropriate testing facilities with informed consent and pre- and post-test counselling.
3. That those who are asymptomatic HIV positive should be enabled to live normal lives in the community, with health care and support based as far as possible on primary care teams in the district of residence.
4. That those who have ARC/AIDS should be managed on a shared-care model used for most chronic, complex disorders and incorporating the concepts of good practice for priority-care groups. They should be suppported as much as possible in the community but require close out-patient supervision and easy access to specialist in-patient facilities. People in the terminal stages should, wherever possible, have the choice of where and with whom they would like to die.
5. To build on the expertise developed within the district and encourage its dissemination to other districts.

At the same time, an operational plan was written quite separately, but it became swamped with financial rather than strategic issues, dominated by the district's overspending. Individuals expended considerable energy at the AIDS Executive complaining that AIDS money was not spent on AIDS facilities.

An operational group was set up to evaluate the numerous bids. Once the operational plan was submitted, it was realised that the Executive could not exert an executive function, despite its title, and that the District General Manager was having the final say on AIDS resource allocation. Moreover, although unit managers had been co-opted on to the AIDS Executive, many decisions taken by the committee were not implemented by them.

The exponential rise in the number of people with AIDS that had occurred until 1986 plateaued within the district during 1987 and, although the cumulative number of cases was rising, there was some easing of the pressure. In addition, the introduction of zidovudine (formerly azidothymidine, or AZT) reduced some of the need for in-patient care. However, it was predicted, based on current referral patterns that there could be over 3,000 cases by 1992 and that patients with AIDS could take up the whole of St Mary's Hospital (Cunningham and Griffiths, 1987). It was agreed by the Executive as part of the strategy that the total number of beds allocated to AIDS should never exceed 56.

The district went through a severe financial crisis at the end of 1987 which delayed the opening of much of the new Queen Elizabeth the Queen Mother wing at St Mary's Hospital. The allocation to the district of large sums of specific funding for AIDS went some way towards relieving this crisis.

1988: The managerial control phase

By mid-1988, managerial control was made explicit for a number of reasons. The district's merger with Brent Health Authority to form Parkside Health Authority required less of a St Mary's-based structure than the AIDS Executive. The merger also created an obvious hiatus when it took some time to fill many managerial posts and funding allocations could not be made. The delays over these allocations created a climate of considerable unrest among those who had submitted bids. Finally, by 1987/8 the scale of AIDS designated money made this funding a significant part of the district's annual budget.

The AIDS Executive formally became an advisory group in July 1988, with executive responsibility passing to the new Acute Services Manager appointed in November 1988. Whether this will clarify executive function remains to be seen. An AIDS co-ordinator, appointed a year earlier to co-ordinate services and liaise with other agencies, became accountable to the Acute Services Manager. Furthermore, the previously agreed post of a specific AIDS Financial Planner, to deal with the increasing costs and availability of funding for AIDS, and the appointment of a GUM Clinic Manager both further confirmed the gradual arrival of AIDS as a major fact of life for the health authority.

The Home Support Team

The Home Support Team is proof of the recognition that AIDS and HIV cannot be managed solely as an acute hospital service. The hospital model of care, with its bias towards short-term treatment ostensibly leaving patients fit enough to return to normal life, is inadequate for people with AIDS. The care necessary for people with HIV and AIDS covers a wide range, from counselling and psycho-social support through to intensive care. The needs of individual patients are likely to be different and each individual's will differ over time. Hospitalisation is only part of the answer.

The practical perception of this problem came from two sources. First, in managerial terms, given St Mary's very wide AIDS catchment area, the hospital care available was inadequate. Second, on the clinical side, there was a perceived need to co-ordinate the hospital service with the fragmented community-based services for patients and their relatives and partners. It was from the acute clinical side that the impetus came, and so, when the Home Support Team was established, managerial responsibility initially went to the clinical immunologist and the manager of in-patient services at St Mary's.

The team was set up in May 1987 and became fully staffed by October 1987, with one co-ordinator (a senior sister with terminal care experience), five nursing sisters, a receptionist and a general practitioner fellow, funded separately by the 'Help the Hospices' charity. The team operates 5 1/2 days a week, always with one person on 24-hour call. The team's broad aim is to co-ordinate hospital and community services, and the team's own stated rationale is

> to initiate an outreach service to give practical care, co-ordinate others and teach by example; to care for patients in their own homes during periods of disability and recovery from acute exacerbations of their illness; to deliver terminal care; and to maintain contact with well patients.

A description of the team's activities, based on nine months of data, elucidated the following facts from the team's records (Victor, 1988). In the first nine months of operation, there were 169 clients on the team's books, of whom 25 died. Eighty-five of the clients were from the hospital (AIDS) ward, with most of the rest coming from the Praed Street Clinic. Only a minority of the clients had a diagnosis of AIDS, although many may have fulfilled the diagnostic criteria. There were considerable nursing care problems because of physical deterioration and incontinence in some patients, but for the majority the difficulties were mostly psycho-social.

The service provided by the team was a combination of telephone contact, home visits and contact at the hospital clinic. Home visits were made to most of the patients who subsequently died as well as to just over half of the others. The nature of the work has been to provide some nursing care, psycho-social support and occasional housing advice or to lobby other agencies. During his year with them, the GP on the team acted to further other GPs' involvement in the care of people with AIDS. This entailed meeting individual GPs, giving seminars, liaising in the care of individual patients, and trying to find GPs prepared to care for patients not registered with one.

How successful the Home Support Team has been in its first year is hotly debated. There have been two related underlying problems. First, there has been an unclear line of managerial control. One consequence of this was the ambiguity of the team's responsibility to patients from within the health district and to those from outside. In general, patient-selection mechanisms were not formally agreed, nor were there clear protocols for referring on to other agencies. Second, there has been little co-ordination with other services at the planning or delivery stage. The district already had district nursing and terminal care services. Although the terminal care service was anxious to keep AIDS at arm's length, it did have the expertise on which the Home Support Team could have drawn in planning its activities, by working on tried concepts of good practice. The district nursing service geared itself up to referrals from the Home Support Team, but these were not forthcoming, perhaps because local patients were quite happy to continue coming to the Wharfside HIV Clinic.

The involvement of other services has been far from universal. Half the clients had no contact with other agencies, and another quarter with just one, usually a GP, social worker or psychologist. There have been difficulties arising from the issue of confidentiality. Clients' privacy has to remain paramount, particularly for those who are not seriously ill, as such people may have far more to lose than to gain from their diagnosis being made available to other agencies. Another problem is that patients come from a wide catchment area which has implications for travel and for liaison with other agencies.

However, these early problems are perhaps being resolved as the Home Support Team enters its second year of activity. They were probably inevitable for any new service within the NHS, particularly one which was set up very quickly, attempting a multi-disciplinary function on its own when there are many other agencies concerned. The plan to bring the Home Support Team under the wing of the community services management now bodes well.

Housing needs

Background
Adequate housing on a short- and long-term basis is a recognised component of community care for people with AIDS and HIV. However, London is at present trying to cope with an increasing number of homeless people. By 1987, 8,000 families had been accepted as 'officially homeless'

(under the 1985 Housing Act), and it is estimated that there are 65,000 single people unofficially homeless in the capital (Association of London Authorities and London Boroughs Association, 1988). In Paddington and North Kensington, the situation is at its worst, with 2,000 families temporarily housed in bed-and-breakfast hotels in the Bayswater area.

The housing requirement for people with HIV or AIDS can arise either because their accommodation is unsuitable for their medical condition or because they are 'homeless'. These two problems can occur in district residents or in those living outside the district but treated at St Mary's (i.e. currently over 75 per cent of HIV/AIDS patients). In addition, there will be those who travel to the district for treatment who may require temporary accommodation.

Accommodation may be unsuitable for a variety of reasons, including:
- access problems if patients' mobility is restricted, and particularly if they are wheelchair-bound.
- dampness and inadequate heating, which is important because of the increased risk of infection in such patients.
- social stigmatisation.

Patients may be homeless because of financial difficulties relating to loss of earnings as a consequence of their ill health or to problems in obtaining mortgages. Some, particularly drug users, may already be homeless as a manifestation of their disordered social lives.

The size of the problem
There are no comprehensive sources of data on the housing status of people with AIDS or HIV infection. The Home Support Team found that 23 (15%) of their first 153 patients had housing problems, 11 because of homelessness and 12 because they lived in unsuitable accommodation (in 5 cases, because of dampness, and difficulties with access in 7). There is also evidence that the problem will worsen as the number of infected drug users who develop symptomatic HIV infection increases, as many of them will lack any social support. Of 61 injecting drug users taking part in the needle exchange scheme (HIV status unknown), 14 (23%) were living in bed-and-breakfast hotels or squats or had no fixed abode.

Current and planned specific housing provision for district patients with HIV and AIDS
Local authorities
In both Westminster (WCC) and Kensington & Chelsea (K&C), decisions about accommodation that is unsuitable on medical grounds are made by their respective medical advisers. This has produced some conflict within K&C because of the predominantly medical nature of the assessment, rather than a multi-disciplinary approach which may be more appropriate.

Those who are homeless must compete with other groups deemed to be 'vulnerable', such as pregnant women, families with children, and the mentally ill. This hierarchical structure means that only those people with HIV-related illness who are most medically unwell are given the greatest priority.

Temporary accommodation – bed and breakfast, private rented or council-owned – is used pending rehousing. Neither local authority has a specific housing strategy relating to HIV/AIDS, but both have AIDS working parties with a housing representative.

Housing associations

Local housing associations are encouraged to develop schemes that cater for groups with special needs such as people with AIDS. However, many proposed schemes have been poorly conceived and are often inappropriate in catering for specific needs. Kensington & Chelsea housing department has produced guidelines for housing associations wishing to provide accommodation specifically for people with HIV or AIDS.

Westminster City Council, with a local church housing association, is currently using 'Housing Corporation' finance, to build a 10-bed unit. Kensington & Chelsea is at present funding one scheme and considering four others. These include an eight-place hostel for those travelling into the area and requiring temporary accommodation, and six cluster flats for those who are either homeless or have unsuitable housing but do not qualify for local authority or housing association accommodation.

The voluntary sector

Turning Point, the voluntary drug agency, is planning to develop a residential facility for drug users with AIDS, particularly for those who continue to use drugs. This is intended to provide a crisis intervention, respite and terminal care facility.

Given the pressure for accommodation in central London, it has been difficult for the health authority to develop its HIV/AIDS strategy, which is seeking to shift the emphasis of care into the community.

A request for a contribution by the health authority to the funding of these schemes – although advocated by the AIDS Executive as it might relieve the pressure on St Mary's – was rejected by management as being within the province of other agencies. The need for full joint planning is understood by most sides but presents intractable practical problems in all multi-agency funding and planning.

London Lighthouse

The London Lighthouse is primarily a hospice run as a charitable foundation. The development of the Lighthouse has been seen as a triumph for the enterprise of a voluntary group headed by Christopher Spence. He and others who were working with Body Positive, the Terrence Higgins Trust and other support groups recognised that care for people with AIDS in the late stages of disease was inadequate, as it was either taking place inappropriately in an acute hospital setting or at home with insufficient support. It was felt that a hospice facility was needed to provide terminal care in a supportive environment.

In 1986, the group approached the district's terminal care service to encourage the development of similar services for AIDS patients, but the terminal care physician did not feel that this was appropriate. As a result, a small London Lighthouse working party set about trying to develop a centre on their own. An empty, run-down old school building in Kensington was earmarked. Initially, there was opposition from local residents, but this was defused after a public meeting and concerted efforts at local public relations. Capital funding was raised from a diverse range of sources including the DHSS, two regional health authorities, London boroughs, charitable donations and trust funds. Several fund-raising activities, such as Ian McKellen's Shakespeare recitals, received much publicity and support, and distinguished people from many walks of life became involved.

Between 1986 and 1988, £4 million capital was raised. The conversion of the building into a well-equipped centre with 24 beds for terminal, respite and convalescent care, and a day area with cafeteria and seminar rooms, was completed in September 1988.

The Lighthouse also runs training programmes for volunteers and statutory health workers, and has a well-organised neighbourhood scheme for providing home care. Medical care is the responsibility of the medical director who previously held the post of general practice facilitator at St Mary's. Some local GPs have been enthusiastic about working on the 24-hour-care rota. Admission and discharge policy aims to maximise the control that clients have over their lives and to minimise the limitations their illness puts on them. Referrals are accepted from clients, carers, GPs and hospitals.

In theory, the centre seems to be a model of its kind, but it remains to be seen what problems develop in practice, particularly how it co-ordinates care with statutory services. It may prove difficult to cater for all categories of people with AIDS and HIV, especially drug users. However, it is a notable achievement and provides a facility not available within the statutory sector.

Female prostitutes

The Praed Street Clinic is one of the main GUM clinics treating prostitutes in central London, and it has a long history of providing regular check-ups for this group of clients. In 1985, a cohort of female prostitutes was recruited from regular attenders to the clinic and from among their contacts. The aim of this study was to investigate the sexual behaviour and lifestyle of prostitutes, particularly in the context of the HIV epidemic. A user-friendly service of regular check-ups on an appointment basis was provided, and results were phoned to the users, which was not standard clinic practice. In return, the users completed a loosely structured questionnaire about sexual behaviour and lifestyle. As a research project, it has been relatively easy to run because it provides a service oriented towards the needs of the prostitutes.

The main problems so far encountered have been the recruitment of drug-using prostitutes and the development of outreach work to increase the size of the cohort. However, the study is now funded by the Medical Research Council, and the aim is to recruit 600 prostitutes, not only from the clinic but also by advertising and by outreach work. This project involves collaboration with other London drug dependency units and GUM clinics treating prostitutes.

The 160 local prostitutes recruited to date are thought to be a fairly representative sample with the exception of drug users. Three prostitutes are known to be HIV antibody positive, but all three have had known high-risk contact: two by sharing dirty needles and one had a boyfriend who was HIV antibody positive. So far, the risk of acquiring HIV infection appears to be from prostitutes' lifestyle while not working rather than from their clients.

The study has shown a high level of safer sex practices with clients, particularly an increase in the use of condoms. The incidence of other sexually transmitted diseases remains low in this cohort, which is also encouraging.

Conclusions

AIDS services in PNK have developed from the interests of specific clinicians, some of whom became national figures in the early days of the response to AIDS. Central government and the regional health authority were informed by and responded to the experience gained in the district, rather than setting the agenda themselves. As AIDS assumed a high national profile, increasing resources were committed to AIDS services.

In contrast to most other district services, which have undergone a period of retraction and rationalisation, AIDS services have mushroomed. The pace of growth has been rapid, and changes have been relatively unplanned. Most have occurred in the acute sector, driven by clinicians' interest and patients' suspicion of primary care and by advances in medical therapy. Management structures have not, until recently, been sufficiently advanced to influence this development significantly or to cope with the increasing bids for specific funding. However, with the growing awareness of AIDS in general and the recognition of the limitations of acute medical care and of the imbalance in service provision, there has been a shift in emphasis towards community care. This did not start easily as it requires considerable inter-agency co-operation and liaison between, on the one hand, primary and community care sectors and, on the other, the acute sector. The problem is compounded in inner London by the geographical distribution of patients between many districts and by the poor match between health authorities' service provision and local authorities' social services. Tighter management structures have been developed and will be needed to co-ordinate and implement service changes proposed in response to the millions of pounds of specific funding for AIDS and the inexorable rise in demand for treatment of people with HIV and AIDS.

At least the first stage of panic response by health care professionals is on the wane.

References

Association of London Authorities and London Boroughs Association. (1988) Working Party on Homelessness. Interim report.

Cunningham, D. and Griffiths, S. F. (1987) AIDS: counting the cost. *British Medical Journal* 295, 921–2.

Department of Environment. (1983) Inner City Directorate. Information Note No. 2: Urban Deprivation London. DoE.

Ferlie, E. and Pettigrew, A. (1988) *The management of change in Paddington and North Kensington DHA: AIDS and acute sector strategy.* Centre for Corporate Strategy and Change, University of Warwick.

Victor, C. (1988) The Paddington and North Kensington AIDS Home Support Team: A description of the first nine months (under review).

HIV Infection in Parkside:
A general practitioner's view

Dr Peter Willis

Being the first and worst affected part of the United Kingdom, all of us working in this area found ourselves 'matriculating in a school for the blind, having our fingers pressed forcibly down on the fiery braille alphabet' of a new and terrifying epidemic that we did not understand. We had only the lessons learned in the United States to guide us, and we largely ignored those because we did not believe that society here was like enough to that in the United States for there to be a problem on anything like the same scale. Besides, in the United States there is no exact equivalent to the British general practitioner from whom we might have gained relevant experience.

First experiences of doctors and patients

Initially, the impact of HIV infection on general practice tended to be very occasional, indiscriminate, sudden and dramatic. There was no consistent pattern: one was unsuspecting, unprepared, often late (sometimes too late) in making the correct diagnosis of HIV infection and generally rather panicked when one did face a probable diagnosis. Patients sensed their doctors' consternation, and the impression was widely disseminated by the gay press that GPs were either rejecting HIV-infected patients or not competent to cope with them. The problem was a new one, a serious one, one for which we did not have a pattern of established responses and – perhaps most alarming of all – one associated with homosexuality, a subject on which many doctors, like most people, have very strong views unillumined by logic or medical science.

Confidentiality of consultations at the GUM clinics became a major issue. General practitioners at first believed themselves to be at risk of infection if they were not informed of their patients' condition, and did not understand the long established principle that GPs were informed of consultations at the clinics only if they had referred the patients or the patients agreed. As doctors learned more about the relatively low infectivity of the virus and the true risks of infection, the possible detrimental effect on the care of the infected patient if the GP is not informed of his or her condition became, and remains, a serious concern.

Confidentiality at the surgery

In the early days, some alarmed GPs were careless about confidentiality and, on occasion, even labelled the outside of patients' record envelopes with their HIV-antibody status. This had disastrous consequences for relationships between people at high risk of infection and their GPs. These events are still widely remembered and are a major obstacle to improving communication between the GUM clinic, patients and their GPs. We did not understand the special nature of HIV infection and its unique impact on patients' lives and environment. Doctors assumed the right to decide for patients whether or not they should have an HIV-antibody test. We now know better, but the widely publicised decision by the BMA Representative Meeting in 1987 to sanction testing without consent was a further setback to gaining the trust of patients.

The widely held view that absolute confidentiality of consultations between patients and their GPs is unlikely remains a major obstacle to providing appropriate care for infected patients. However, the generalisation that HIV-infected patients are unhappy with their GPs has been refuted by several surveys. The fact that the majority of patients who confide in their GPs are very satisfied is something that needs to be made more widely known. Surveys of GPs indicate that most have quietly and competently taken up the challenge and are caring for the infected patients on their lists.

Education for general practitioners

Until a few years ago, we had had no education about HIV infection. We had left medical school with no inkling of it and often with little modern understanding of immunology. The staff at the GUM clinics, who had all the experience, were overwhelmed by their work caring for patients with HIV-related disease, calming the anxieties of their hospital colleagues and answering the questions thrown at them by the press. Patients went direct to the GUM clinics, and the GP was left isolated with a false impression of the rarity of the infection. When ill patients presented in the surgery, we were thus completely unprepared. It is perhaps not surprising that on a number of occasions the response was inappropriate. Those with specialist knowledge of HIV infection now realise the importance of spreading their knowledge efficiently by training key health workers. GPs working in the community will be particularly important as the burden of everyday care of infected people becomes too great for hospital-based doctors to cope with. A well-prepared GP is far more likely to react appropriately to the vast array of problems – medical and social – that HIV infection may produce.

Educational meetings for general practitioners laid a good foundation, especially when a GP and a person with HIV infection were included among the speakers. The former is the only person who can relate the information to the realities of general practice, and the latter is the only person who can relate the reality of being infected to those who are uninfected. Watching a health adviser role-playing a counselling session has been an extremely illuminating experience for GPs who, traditionally, have a more directive style of guidance. However, individual patients and their problems are an excellent basis for learning in general practice. Perhaps the best form of learning occurs when patients are discharged from hospital to the care of their GPs backed up by the Home Support Team, who can provide all the information, support, advice and care that is appropriate both for the patient and the primary health care team. Time spent on relatively few patients should pay dividends as, in this way, GPs and their teams gain confidence and need progressively less support.

General practitioners and the hospital

Communication between GPs and the hospital when patients are discharged remains a troublesome problem. The tradition of confidentiality, together with the escalating clinical workload in a speciality that is unfamiliar with the procedures of a well-arranged discharge to the primary health care team, has led to a still inadequately resolved problem. It is very bad for professional relationships when the GP is called to a recently discharged and gravely ill patient on a Saturday night with no idea that he or she has ever been in hospital. Instead of the GP learning from the experience, he or she may have unhelpful feelings of resentment.

The understandable reasons why HIV-infected people wish to have absolute confidentiality become relatively insignificant when they become ill. There is a great need for improvement in communication about ill patients between specialist and GP for the benefit of all concerned. When the reasons for involving their GPs are explained adequately, most patients will agree to this in order to ensure the best possible care. At a somewhat earlier stage, before there is any serious illness, record cards carried by patients (thereby avoiding the need for written records in their GPs' notes) would greatly facilitate communication of information which patients might otherwise not allow.

General practitioners and their teams

General practitioners who are themselves dealing confidently with HIV-infected patients are able to allay the anxieties which other members of the primary care team may be experiencing. Demonstrating confidentiality, compassion, care and absence of fear is the best possible reassurance to those who have had less opportunity to gain confidence. In addition, specific time set aside for staff to meet and discuss their fears and to ask questions is helpful in avoiding panic. Receptionists should be included in these arrangements as they have even fewer opportunities than other health workers to discuss their feelings.

Home-helps are crucial to the ability of many people to stay at home, and they also need to be educated and supported. We have learned that the family of the home-help may also need to be considered when explaining the negligible risk of HIV infection in domestic situations. The recruitment of home-helps specifically for this work may be helpful initially, but it is probably wrong in the long term to imply that only specially selected people can care for people with AIDS.

New relationships between doctor and patient

HIV infection has brought about a change in the relationship between general practitioner and patient. Our patients may know more about their infection and treatment than we do ourselves. They certainly want to know in detail what is happening to them and expect to be involved in decisions about their treatment in a way which is quite new. This may shock some GPs, but it is also refreshing. Far from coming to the doctor with blind faith that the doctor will somehow take on the responsibility for making them better, patients come for support in shouldering the burden themselves. We find ourselves one of a range of people sharing in this support. We may become very important and respected advisers, but we are less likely to be the star players that we traditionally expect to be. Occasionally patients come to us feeling very anxious or frightened and needing a confident, parent-figure doctor; but the doctor must then be prepared to revert to being comrade-in-arms or whipping-boy as their needs change. Fulfilling these different roles is not easy for the general practitioner. Doctors and patients may gain comfort from sharing the burdens created by the disease, but the truth is that, with the current state of knowledge, doctors cannot make their patients better in the long run, and that what both are striving for is the best possible health and the best possible life for an uncertain length of time.

The Bloomsbury Response to HIV and AIDS

Dr Rob George and Dr Graham Hart

Setting the scene

Bloomsbury Health Authority ostensibly serves a population of 130,000 in north and central London, from Soho in the south to St John's Wood in the north. Yet with an annual budget of £120 million, and employing over 8,000 people, the authority is typical of districts in central and inner London in that its 'true' population includes people living outside the area but selectively using its specialist services. 'Bloomsbury' was created in 1982, and two of the 19 hospitals inherited at that time were University College Hospital (UCH) and the Middlesex, both major teaching hospitals enjoying national and international reputations. Many developments within the district in relation to AIDS have benefited from the interaction of NHS and academic departments.

Socially, economically and politically diverse, both Bloomsbury's resident population and the larger constituency it serves include many members of two of the historical high-risk groups for HIV infection – namely, homosexual/bisexual men and injecting drug users. Indeed, many features of the history of the epidemic in the district match the larger history of the epidemic in this country, with the first cases of AIDS appearing in the homosexual community.

Table 3 shows the total number of AIDS reports from the district between 1983 and mid-1988; gay men constitute the majority of cases throughout. Antibody testing for HIV began early in 1985 using the world's first HIV antibody test, devised by the Department of Virology at the Middlesex Hospital. Up to May 1988, 707 positive test results had been identified.

Homosexual and bisexual men

Since the early 1970s, a feature of the lifestyles of many homosexual and bisexual men in London has been increased opportunities for sexual activity with multiple partners. One unintended but natural consequence of this has been a high incidence of sexually transmitted diseases (STDs) among gay men; as a result, attendance at STD clinics increased throughout the 1970s and early 1980s.

In Bloomsbury, open-access genito-urinary medicine (GUM) clinics are available at major teaching hospitals. James Pringle House (JPH) at the Middlesex Hospital is the second largest GUM clinic in the UK, with an

Table 3 **AIDS reports to CDSC from Bloomsbury Health District 1983–8**

| | Reported to CDSC | | Known to have died | |
	Number	Cumulative total	Number	Cumulative total
1983	3	3	2	2
1984	11	14	4	6
1985	20	34	9	15
1986	33	67	22	37
1987	63	130	40	77
Jan–June 1988	27	157	20	97

annual total of 70,000 attendances. It is physically separate from the main hospital – on Charlotte Street, W1 – and its central location and the non-judgemental attitude of the staff have made it popular with gay men.

This clinic also houses the Academic Department of Genito-urinary Medicine. When this was founded in 1979, it comprised a clinical chair, a clinical lectureship and two supporting staff but, by 1988, this had grown to a multi-disciplinary staff of more than 30, mainly funded by research grants. Early in the epidemic, senior members of the Department, taking note of the developing situation in the United States, were quick to establish research projects and argue for services to be provided. At first, this could only be on the basis of a few people with AIDS as no seroprevalence data were available but, by 1986, research showed that 25 per cent of the gay men who attended the clinic were HIV-antibody positive. This prevalence of infection – approximately 1 in 4 of the 5,000 gay men attending the clinic – has remained constant since then (Carne *et al.*, 1986).

Injecting drug users

North and central London has one of the highest concentrations of injecting drug users in the capital. Bloomsbury has a drug dependency clinic at the National Temperance Hospital which serves this population. Awareness of the potential spread of HIV among drug users, and beyond to the heterosexual population, began to increase in 1985/6, partly in response to American epidemiology and partly to data coming from Scotland (Des

Jarlais and Friedman, 1987; Robertson *et al.*, 1986).

Some movement on this issue took place in 1985 when a new Senior Lecturer in Psychiatry was appointed, with sessions at the drug clinic. Her concern about the problem was shared by some of the workers at the drug dependency clinic, and this led to a close collaboration with staff at JPH for a combination of service and research. A study undertaken in 1986/7 indicated an HIV-antibody positive rate of 4 per cent in drug users attending the clinic, and considerable potential for prevention (Hart, Sonnex *et al.*, 1989).

The local response

The Professor of Genito-urinary Medicine played an important role in putting AIDS on the health agenda of the country as a whole. The majority of cases of AIDS, and subsequently of HIV infection, in Bloomsbury presented initially at JPH, and from 1983 the academic department was in the forefront of demands for adequate services. This was not simply for increased medical personnel at JPH, but for a comprehensive service based in the out-patient department, the hospital, the laboratory and the community.

Funding for services
In April 1985, bids for DHSS funds were submitted to the regional health authority for a dedicated AIDS ward, the development of JPH's out-patient department, improved testing facilities and a dedicated facility for people with HIV-related disease at the Dental Hospital.

The decision (in October 1985) to allocate only £275,000 to the district meant that not all of these proposals could be financed. There was even a management proposal that these monies should be used to reduce the district's overspending, but this suggestion was determinedly opposed by a coalition of interested individuals who lobbied the health authority and the DHSS, before a final ruling was made against the management proposal. Decisions as to how to spend the allocation were therefore passed to a specialist committee which, by no accident, included the key contributors in the formulation of the bids and whose firm commitment was to service development.

Over the next two years, this committee – described elsewhere (Ferlie and Pettigrew, 1988) as the 'kitchen cabinet' – was to play a major role in allocating resources and producing further bids. At first (1985/6), it put proposals to the District General Manager and the District Management Board whence they were referred to the health authority for formal approval. This was, for the most part, a series of formalities as the expert views of the 'kitchen cabinet' were more often than not accepted by senior management.

Figure 3 **Organisation structures 1985–6 (after Ferlie and Pettigrew, 1988)**

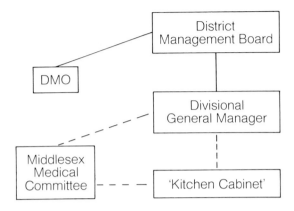

Thus, by 1987, the Middlesex had its own dedicated AIDS ward, ending the previously fragmented in-patient care. This was a major achievement which had necessitated the lobbying and persuasion of powerful forces within the hospital who opposed and resisted such a development. JPH had successfully undertaken new building work and, along with some refurbishment, had substantially extended its counselling and out-patient facilities. Indeed, by 1988, all of the proposals of the 1985 bid had finally been realised.

A structure for community services

All of the services described so far are essentially hospital based. However, the interests of the Professor of Genito-urinary Medicine, the District Medical Officer and the Lecturer in Epidemiology – all members of the 'kitchen cabinet' – were much broader, and efforts to widen the scope of services were a key feature of developments from 1986 onwards. There was interest in the possible benefits of health outreach programmes and primary health care and home care teams, and increasingly vocal demands for support from the drug dependency clinic. It was clear that the 'kitchen cabinet' should be augmented by the AIDS Steering Committee and, in 1986, a group representing wider interests was set up to take recommendations from the 'kitchen cabinet' and to make decisions. It included a wide range of people, including representatives from the local social services departments and a GP.

The number of staff and committees undertaking AIDS- or HIV-related work was increasing. In 1987, an AIDS co-ordinator was appointed to make connections between the disparate sections of the AIDS system, identify gaps, encourage liaison and ensure that proposals and allocations were compatible.

By April 1987, the district allocation was only £300,000 short of what had been requested, and the profile of Bloomsbury's response to AIDS was

Figure 4 **Organisation structures 1987–8 (after Ferlie and Pettigrew, 1988)**

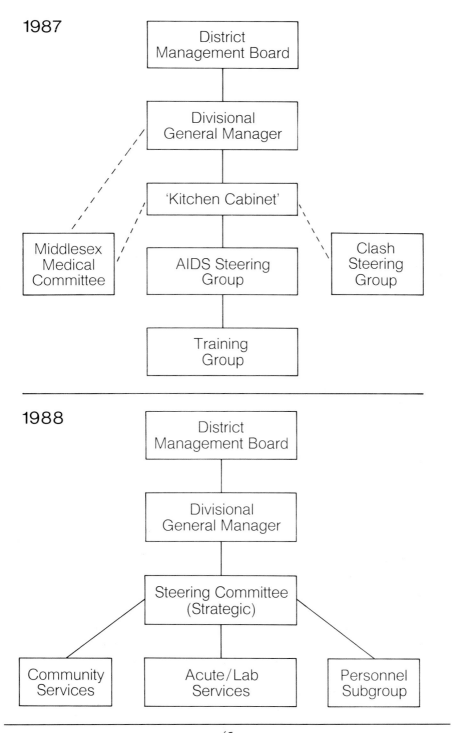

clearly discernible. From a firm hospital base in the form of the AIDS ward and, at JPH, the open access to primary and preventive care for anyone concerned about HIV infection as well as for users at the drug dependency clinic, the strategy became increasingly outward looking and community oriented. The development of two of these approaches is described below in more detail: the Community Care Team and the strategy for drug users.

Of course, there were, and still are, gaps in services. For example, there has been only limited success in encouraging local GPs to take responsibility for the care of people with HIV-related disease. Although a self-selected and highly motivated group of GPs are involved, they are by no means representative of all the local ones, and it has proved particularly difficult to involve GPs in the formal planning process. Similarly, liaison with the two local authorities of which Bloomsbury is part (Camden and Westminster) has not been easy, often because of the pressures on inner city social services departments, but partly because of the lack of coterminosity with district boundaries.

In a review such as this, space does not allow for more than a cursory analysis of events and processes, especially when this has been undertaken so competently elsewhere (Ferlie and Pettigrew, 1988). What is missing is a full account of the bitter and occasionally acrimonious disputes and battles within and between specialities, management, staff at all levels, and district and region health authorities, and the politics, lobbying and 'horse trading' which are so much a feature of AIDS-related work.

In one way, this is a positive omission as it avoids the undue weight sometimes placed on individuals, and the rarely appropriate casting of people as heroes or villains (*cf.* Shilts, 1988). More frequently, people reflect perspectives resulting from professional judgment, or they express dominant social concerns, rather than views that are idiosyncratic or in some way peculiar.

The next section allows us to focus in greater detail on two features of service provision which are concerned with opposite ends of the HIV spectrum. The drug-related services try to help drug users avoid infection, and the Community Care Team aims to help people die with dignity in surroundings of their choice.

Services for drug users

Statutory services for drug users in the district are split three ways, and this account will follow that division. These are the drug dependency clinic, the needle exchange scheme and the health outreach programme. The focus here is on statutory provision, but all three services interact and liaise with voluntary agencies within and outside the district as appropriate.

The drug dependency clinic

Bloomsbury's drug dependency clinic at the National Temperance Hospital serves an area with one of the largest concentrations of drug users in the capital.

In the late 1960s and early 1970s, the clinic offered injectable heroin and Methadone – usually as a reducing prescription, but sometimes involving long-term or maintenance prescribing. However, by the early 1980s, most injecting drug users were offered oral Methadone on a rapidly reducing prescription, together with a treatment package which could include psychotherapy, group work, counselling and teaching on life-skills.

This was the essential philosophy of drug dependency units and of the psychiatrists working within them at that time – i.e. a situation where the addict eventually becomes drug free via an integrated approach within which Methadone plays a major role. For some workers, the appearance of HIV infection in their treatment population resulted in a questioning of this philosophy; for others, it was an affirmation of its value. This example of opposing philosophies will be discussed later.

Identifying the need

Reports from the United States, Europe and Scotland indicating a high prevalence of HIV infection among drug users led to concern as to the nature of the service offered to clients at the drug dependency clinic. At the same time, the Academic Department of Genito-urinary Medicine became interested in the extension of the HIV epidemic to and beyond a primarily heterosexual population of drug users. In 1986, a series of joint meetings between both departments led to an agreement that a combined research and primary health care service be offered to users, initially for a period of one year.

Although the drug dependency clinic had been offering AIDS health education in the form of group sessions, leaflets and posters, staff soon saw the benefit of a primary health service which provided screening for hepatitis B infection, skin and systemic disease, along with advice on contraception, pregnancy and nutrition. With opportunities for counselling and testing for HIV infection as an integral part of the service, the team of a clinician and nurse were able to encourage perception of the service in terms of the promotion of overall physical and psychological health, without undue emphasis on the risk of HIV-related disease.

The study associated with the service (Hart, Sonnex *et al.*, 1989) found a prevalence of HIV infection in 108 clients, or 4 per cent, although evidence of previous hepatitis B infection was found in the sera of 64 per cent, clearly indicating previous high-risk behaviour for blood borne viral infections. Indeed, 87 per cent of the clients had shared needles and syringes at some point in their drug-using history, and of these 75 per cent had shared within the previous year, usually with friends or sexual partners.

Clients were asked about behaviour change since the appearance of

AIDS. While the majority (62%) had made some positive change in their drug using behaviour, only 31 per cent had adopted safer sexual practices. This undoubtedly reflects some success on the part of health education efforts within and outside the drug dependency clinic, but clearly indicated the potential scope for further behavioural change.

The Health Improvement Team

After one year, members of the health assessment team from James Pringle House were required to fulfil other duties, which meant that the service had to cease temporarily. However, by this time an application for further funding had been successful and, from November 1987, a clinician, psychologist and two nurses were recruited to join the new Health Improvement Team (HIT).

As there has not yet been enough time to evaluate the HIT, it is worth identifying some of the positive and negative aspects of the services provided by the first health assessment team.

Apart from the immediate health care benefits of assessment – such as referral to specialist hospital departments – the presence of a GU physician experienced in HIV infection meant that long-term physical and psychological care of HIV-antibody-positive users could be offered at James Pringle House, with access to the dedicated AIDS ward in the Middlesex Hospital. For all clients, regardless of antibody status, the counselling and advice provided by the team nurse introduced or reinforced health education. In addition, the data collected provided valuable measures of risky behaviour and provided a baseline for future studies.

As the assessment was offered only on one day each week, many appointments were broken. With the full-time Health Improvement Team, compliance may increase, particularly if drug assessments or prescriptions are arranged for the same day.

Provision of this type of primary health care has, for the most part, been welcomed by a group whose contact with health services has often been fraught with difficulties. Drug dependency units and other psychiatric-based services for drug users might usefully consider this more rounded model of patient care.

The needle exchange scheme

In response to requests from injecting drug users attending the casualty department at UCH, a service began in Bloomsbury in January 1987 to exchange sterile needles and syringes for used ones. The drug and alcohol advisory nurse took responsibility for this service which, within a short time, was seeing over 200 clients a month.

At that time, no evaluation of needle exchange schemes had been undertaken in this country, to see if they could realise their primary goal – the prevention of HIV infection. When it became clear in the spring of 1987 that the government was interested in supporting a number of needle exchange schemes, a strong case was made to the DHSS to fund two workers. This was agreed on condition that the scheme formed part of a national evaluation. It was felt that local evaluation, including voluntary antibody testing, could contribute substantially to knowledge in this area. The AIDS Virus and Education Research Trust (AVERT) supported this, and acceded to a proposal for a two-year research assistant post.

As the scheme was proving popular with drug users, and numbers were increasing monthly, the extra burden that the service was placing on an already over-stretched casualty department was unacceptable. To overcome this, the planned move of the Middlesex Hospital's Department of Surgical Appliances from a shop-fronted building separate from the main hospital was expedited, and the needle exchange transferred from the UCH casualty department to 16A Cleveland Street in September 1987.

Although by no means perfect, the newly decorated and refurbished offices, with their own entrance and central location, soon proved popular. This was in no small part due to the efforts of the two drug and health education workers who, five days every week, provide needles and syringes on an exchange basis, as well as sterile water and condoms. They also offer advice on suitable injecting sites, and other harm-reduction techniques, along with limited primary health care such as dressings for abscesses and referral to the casualty department when indicated.

Although the needle exchange is clearly not a drug treatment agency since it facilitates safer drug use, it is in close contact with and often makes referrals to voluntary drug agencies in the area, including a crisis centre and street agencies concerned with the welfare of drug users. Other referrals go to a local GP, who is willing to take a small number of patients on a month's Methadone reduction programme, and to the drug dependency clinic.

By January 1988, the primary nursing care offered in the exchange was supplemented by the availability, on site, of physicians two afternoons every week for consultation on a wide range of health concerns.

Evaluation

Local evaluation of the scheme offers evidence of its popularity (Hart, Carvell *et al.*, 1988). Between January and December 1988, the average number of clients attending every month was 273, each making an average of approximately three visits per month. The majority of clients were male (male:female = 4:1) with a mean age of 32, and mean daily injecting drug history of 14 years.

Figure 5 shows the number of syringes dispensed and returned during this 12-month period, with a variable return rate which averages 80 per cent. A representative sample (n=94) of all attenders reported a low prevalence of sharing, with 80 per cent having neither borrowed nor lent injecting equipment one month after entry into the scheme. However, the majority of people had shared within the previous two years, indicating earlier risky behaviour. With an HIV-antibody-positive prevalence of 9 per

Figure 5 **Syringe return rate, January to December 1988**

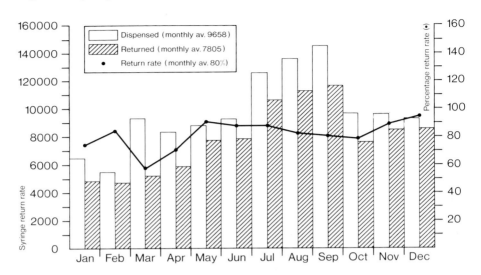

cent in this population, the health education work of the needle exchange must continue, alongside the provision of sterile injecting equipment.

The needle exchange in Bloomsbury – popular with users and enjoying a high client return rate – also, according to the staff, sees fewer episodes of injecting-related morbidity, such as abscesses and septicaemia. Fifty per cent of clients report regular use of condoms which is much higher than in comparable primarily heterosexual populations.

While commercial pharmacies may be able to facilitate increased availability of needles and syringes, they are not usually able to offer clients any other services, including referral to treatment agencies, primary health care or help and advice. Increased availability of injecting equipment should be encouraged, but this should ideally take place in the context of comprehensive health provision.

Problems

These are confined to administration rather than service. One consequence of receiving initial funding from outside the district was the failure to establish a clear delineation of management. The interdisciplinary steering group proved unable to meet the challenge of the daily management of a busy project and this was reflected in the fact that one worker handed in his notice after three months because of the undue strain. Long hours in a stressful occupation without adequate financial and managerial support is clearly a recipe for low staff morale. This event, among others, contributed to the subsequent reorganisation into a greatly improved management structure. The needle exchange is now under the aegis of the Bloomsbury Mental Health Unit, with a commitment from the district to continue funding and increase staffing.

Tensions in philosophy

The primary philosophy of the agency may have both positive and negative consequences. For example, the strategy to facilitate safer needle use is supported by all of the voluntary agencies with which the scheme liaises, and results in extremely good working relationships. However, some professionals within the statutory sector are either lukewarm about it or are overtly antipathetic to it. This also applies to strong client advocacy which has long been a feature of voluntary drug agency strategy but not necessarily a feature of statutory service provision. It is no surprise that the needle exchange, enjoying a degree of autonomy not usually found in the health service, has adopted to some extent a voluntary agency perspective.

While this has not resulted in open conflict between the needle exchange and statutory services, tensions have existed in their working relationship. Clinic workers have worked for many years with a model of care which emphasised abstinence rather than harm reduction, and abstinence by definition cannot countenance the facilitation of safer use of street drugs.

Fortunately, close contact and regular meetings between the two staffs have resulted in greater flexibility. While the dominant philosophy of the drug dependency clinic has been towards abstinence, it does have a number of drug users on Methadone maintenance. The needle exchange workers will also help clients who wish to end their dependency, including a referral to the clinic, waiting lists permitting. However, the potential for major conflicts in other districts is one that should be recognised before services such as needle exchanges are set up. These are not clashes of personality, but of working philosophies; such differences, however, need not be irreconcilable.

The health outreach programme

The recognition in that some groups in the population are not in contact with or are actually excluded from primary health care services because of their lifestyles has led to a questioning of well-established models of service provision. Rather than making a service available and then expecting people to come forward, without any regard to cultural context or the practical realities of their daily lives, greater efforts have been made in the direction of health outreach work. Now firmly established in the drugs field, this is an example of a service which seeks out potential clients, using social networks to educate, inform and promote health.

Central London attracts a large indigent population of young people, many of whom are unemployed and homeless. Some are on the fringes of a drug-using sub-culture, and others may exchange sex for money, food or shelter. It is clear that many young people in this situation are at risk of blood-borne and sexually transmitted infections such as HIV.

With this in mind, talks between staff in the Academic Department of Genito-urinary Medicine and voluntary organisations in the West End began as early as November 1985 around the issue of health promotion for young people at risk in central London. Although the motivating concern was prevention and control of HIV infection, other sexually transmitted diseases, drug use and primary health care were all on the agenda. A bid to fund a health outreach team was successful in July 1986 and, by the end of the year, three workers were in their posts. Central London Action on Street Health (CLASH) began work as a local outreach programme targeting young people.

Once again, it was considered vital to evaluate the work of this initiative, and a joint proposal with the Drug Indicators Project (DIP) at Birkbeck College was approved by the DHSS. A research assistant has been in post since March 1988, working from DIP.

It is too early to report on the progress of the research, but on the positive side CLASH does seem to be reaching members of its target population. One of the workers, for example, has made a particular effort to contact male prostitutes ('rent boys') on the street and in pubs and clubs, distributing condoms and talking about safer sex. Other workers have contacted female prostitutes working from flats in Soho and on the streets in the King's Cross area. The CLASH workers also provide an informal health promotion service to voluntary and statutory agencies serving drug users in the West End.

It is difficult to identify negative features at this early stage. Because of the inherently delicate nature of much outreach work (drug users' and prostitutes' associations with illegal activities), the scheme took some time before it was fully operational. Ensuring that one is acceptable to these groups, and not associated in any way with the criminal justice system, is a time-consuming and sensitive process. It also took some time for the workers to establish themselves with professionals working in both the voluntary and statutory sectors. To do this, they emphasised the potential value of the service, avoided possibly damaging 'territorial' disputes and liaised in such a way as to ensure that referrals of individuals by CLASH workers were met with an appropriate response from service providers.

Although at first coming under the auspices of 'health education', the workers found that many of the skills they required were those of counselling and the provision of advice, and so their management was transferred to the Principal Clinical Psychologist at James Pringle House. As time moves on, it may be found that another structural location will be required, perhaps related to other complementary services such as HIT, the needle exchange and the Community Care Team (described below). This is an expression of the difficulties associated with pressing new service developments into old service structures, a feature of much AIDS-related provision. With its multi-disciplinary demands, the prevention and treatment of HIV disease requires formal communication networks between different departments, and may require the introduction of integrated units. Simply employing a single 'AIDS co-ordinator' is not necessarily the answer to these problems.

Summary of drug services

It has been necessary for the purposes of this account to describe separately each of these services – HIT, the needle exchange and CLASH. This is partly to ensure clarity, but also because each service has its own history within the broad model of service provision in Bloomsbury. However, what should be emphasised is that close liaison, referrals from and joint working between the three projects are central to their respective activities.

All of the projects enjoy good relations with voluntary agencies locally, and this applies particularly to CLASH and the needle exchange workers. Apart from being good working practice, this has occurred partly because these two schemes are undertaking work more usually associated with the voluntary sector, and indeed many project staff have previous experience of working for voluntary agencies.

From this account, it is clear that Bloomsbury is offering a reasonably integrated, if not yet fully comprehensive, service to injecting drug users in relation to health promotion in general and HIV infection in particular. Yet the three services that combine to realise this health strategy have had, and will continue to experience, problems, both in terms of the practicalities of daily work and in connecting with and complementing other services in the district. Other districts would be well advised to consider in detail the nature of their local situation before adopting strategies which may well prove to be Bloomsbury-specific.

The Bloomsbury Community Care Team (BCCT)

History

While Bloomsbury opened one of the first dedicated in-patient facilities in the UK for people with AIDS, it has also been in the vanguard of community-based initiatives for this client group, some of which have been described above. At the end of 1986, attention began to turn to the long-term provision for people with increasing disability as they approached death, and the subject of community and 'terminal' care therefore arose. At that stage, however, following Norman Fowler's visit to San Francisco, thought was inclining more towards the need for hospice facilities rather than continuing care within the home.

In addition, an increasing number of patients were flowing through the new dedicated ward and were developing strong links with that facility. This was continuing when they returned home, either by telephone contact or by early self-referral back into the system. While this would ordinarily have been the remit of the GPs and primary health care teams, many clients had preconceptions of general practice that made them wary of this system. This naturally led to the ward extending its remit to that of respite and terminal care, and the historic tendency of STD clinics to provide primary care independent of the GPs was reinforced.

With the excellent out-patient reputation of James Pringle House, the most logical solution was to develop some HIV-dedicated service linking the ward, clinic and community services. Informal discussions with a number of people with AIDS confirmed that the overriding need in the provision of continuing care or symptom palliation was to help people within their own homes, backed up by appropriate terminal care or respite facilities. Apparently no other centre was addressing this area, so there was clearly a need either to adapt or to create an alternative approach.

In March 1987, one of the hospital physicians involved in in-patient care submitted a preliminary proposal for a community-based multi-disciplinary team. The development and process of this initiative is summarised below, together with comments and suggestions of how high- and low-prevalence areas might use our experience.

Was there an existing model from which to learn?
The Bloomsbury Cancer Home Support Team
Many districts in the UK have home care teams looking after people with cancer, and the most effective of these have a multi-disciplinary approach. Within Bloomsbury, a multi-disciplinary home care team already had five years' experience catering for the needs of those dying of cancer at home. They function largely as advisers to existing services.

It was evident at a very early stage that extension of this team into AIDS-related work would not be feasible for two principal reasons, independent of the specific issues related to HIV and AIDS.

(1) Their remit was restricted to Bloomsbury, but only 10–20 per cent of the HIV client group are resident within the district.

(2) There was concern about team dynamic. It is widely accepted within terminal care that teams exceeding eight members, particularly if there are more than four clinicians (nurses and/or doctors), are at risk of poor communication. The cancer team was already working at full capacity and wished to remain small.

While the size of the AIDS problem in Bloomsbury is sufficient to sustain the development of a dedicated team, this is unlikely to be the case in areas of low prevalence, where an appropriate but limited expansion of existing services would be in the interests of both staff and patients (*see below*).

In Bloomsbury, the proposal was based largely upon the wheel that had already been invented. This had two advantages; it seemed the most appropriate way of approaching the problem and it was already an existing and accepted model within the health district.

The proposal

This incorporated a statement of the general philosophical approach to community and palliative care and management of people with AIDS through death, together with an outline of the research that might come out of such a venture. With the establishment and maturing of the project the ways of working out these ideas have become clearer.

Philosophy of care

This initiative began at a time when there was little or no concrete experience of 'terminal care' for people with AIDS. However, the basic principle of care for whatever client group approaching death is essentially to move from interventionist diagnostic and therapeutic medicine towards a more pragmatic approach which is patient-driven and incorporates issues outside the conventional remit of clinical medicine. There is an emphasis on aspects of symptom control and on resolution of the issues relating to death and dying, together with a clear sense of control remaining with the patient.

While there is nothing new in this global management of individuals within the context of their lives, and the needs of those dying young are common to all diseases, these needs are compounded by the cultural and social implications of HIV and AIDS. This has tended to make palliative and terminal care in AIDS a relatively specialised and evolving area. For example, the notion of there being a clear and predictable 'terminal phase' in HIV-related disease is unfounded. Thus the application of 'terminal care' philosophy and practice, while pertinent, is particularly fluid at the moment. This is especially evident with respect to the definition of symptom control and the grey area between active and palliative care.

Integration with existing statutory or voluntary services

Any service wishing to help people through this phase of their lives should be able to create or facilitate a person's environment and support system within the community or within dedicated facilities. Many of the individual needs of clients are well fulfilled by statutory services which already exist, either within primary health care or a local authority. These are matched by the major and highly organised voluntary inputs that are available. It seemed clear then that the role of the Community Care Team should be to facilitate, integrate, enable and support the work already being done within both the voluntary and statutory sectors, rather than create another complete layer of care provision. It was therefore recognised at an early stage that there should be close and ongoing links between the team and a variety of agencies.

Education and advice

The Team would take on a measure of responsibility for information, education and training of primary health care services as appropriate. BCCT would also be available to advise on symptom control and specialist care needs as a patient approached death, and would provide an appropriate diagnostic service should the need arise.

'Hands-on care'

The degree to which the team should provide a direct clinical service to a person with AIDS was difficult to predict. This certainly seemed an area in which the BCCT could differ from the clear advisory role of the cancer team. The ideal in a sense would be to disseminate and devolve clinical expertise and responsibility to the primary health care teams and general home care teams so that, with the passage of time, the role of the specialist team would either be defunct or more concentrated on the specific needs of the indigenous Bloomsbury population. A year on, there is little doubt that a specific 'HIV team' will be needed for some time to come.

Evaluation and research

The home-care team for cancer already had an established research link with the Department of Community Medicine in University College London (UCL). This work, under the supervision of Mark McCarthy, had a validated and effective multi-centre evaluation programme looking at the impact of cancer home care teams upon symptom control and quality of life, as well as their effectiveness as perceived by client and family.

For a rapid means of establishing evaluation and an unique opportunity to compare palliative care of people with AIDS and cancer, it seemed logical to adopt this schedule as the bedrock of team audit.

Apart from the adaptation of the existing UCL evaluation programme, the Team was expecting to provide data on patterns of disease process, the appropriateness of certain therapeutic interventions and an estimate of practical care needs, together with the projection of expected needs in the future. These descriptive data are urgently needed.

Team structure

Initial modelling would be one full-time physician at senior lecturer level with two full-time specialist nurse practitioners – one in community nursing and one in terminal care – as well as a social worker with particular skills in the care of those approaching death, a full-time researcher to run evaluation programmes and an administrator. It was felt that the appointment of a physician should be at consultant level, and that all team members should have established pedigrees in their areas of speciality to give credibility and momentum to this venture.

Initial Team brief

Service to the patient   The objective was to provide choice for the patient and 'family' between continuing care at hospital, at home or in appropriate hospice facilities. This was to be achieved by providing an integration between hospital and statutory community services and the voluntary sector.

Service to other health care professionals   In situations where existing services were inadequate or failing, the Team was to provide hands-on care if appropriate. However, wherever possible, clinical responsibility was to be placed firmly with the general practitioner and primary health care team.

Local authorities and other agencies would be expected to contribute to home support in ways similar to those for other client groups.

Implementation

The initiative was welcomed in principle by senior medical staff in the departments of medicine, and departments of genito-urinary medicine, where there was already close co-operation on in-patient and out-patient care. Very active support from the Bloomsbury Community Unit management gave significant impetus to the venture. Following refinements to the project, funding was made available: approximately one-third from district, a single grant from the King's Fund and the remainder from the Monument Trust. The senior lecturer entered post in December 1987, and the rest of the team began in April 1988.

In these first months, the essential groundwork and networking was begun in close association with the existing provisions within Bloomsbury and with the wider networks of voluntary and statutory community services across the metropolis. For example, links were forged with key people in the hospice movement. The senior lecturer was also on the consultant staff of the Mildmay Continuing Care Unit for AIDS since its inception as the first residential unit of this type to open in Europe.

These early contacts were fundamental to the subsequent success and acceptability of the team. Colleagues needed the opportunity to acclimatise to the notion of another agency making a contribution towards alleviating the complex array of medical, nursing and social needs. For instance, within the Middlesex Hospital, the ward's role had extended to meet some of the needs for continuing care, hospital clinicians were being used as GPs, and health advisers were fulfilling many aspects normally met by social workers. Within the community, there was very little evidence, at least as far as many primary health care teams were concerned, that AIDS was a problem. This was coupled paradoxically with anxiety that the existence of a team would undermine primary health care. This 'softly softly approach' certainly minimised some of the territorial issues that would inevitably arise. A limited but flexible clinical service was initially provided by the senior lecturer to explore the areas of potential weakness and conflict.

While this slightly surreptitious start had early advantages, the rapid accumulation of clients soon helped the Team to develop more robust and concrete ideas of their role that were not open to easy manipulation. There were one or two abrasions. In fact, the starting point in many Team meetings on role was usually a statement of what we did *not* see as our function. However, a firm commitment to succeed and a proactive approach to interdisciplinary problems has minimised blood loss.

The development of the 'Team role'

There were four clear areas where problems were likely to be encountered: the interaction between ward, out-patients and the Team; the wide geographical spread of patients; the apparent resistance of patients to their GPs being involved in hands-on care within the community; and the wide spectrum of care structures surrounding individuals rather than the more 'conventional' small family units that are seen more often in the context of people dying with cancer.

Interactions between the Team and the hospital

The Team is based at the National Temperance Hospital and is therefore seen as being discrete from other hospital-based services. This choice was forced by the need for accommodation, but it has proved useful as a way of reinforcing the Team's separate identity.

The formalised interactions are shown most clearly in Figure 6. The hub of communication is formed by the weekly multi-disciplinary ward meeting where in-patient referrals are made and discharges planned.

Figure 6 Interaction between Bloomsbury clinical services

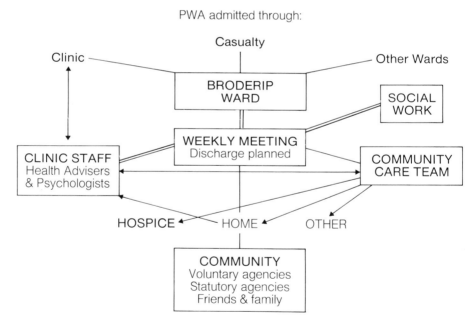

The senior lecturer is a general and chest physician in both the Academic Departments of Medicine and Genito-urinary Medicine. This fact has reassured both patients and hospital staff that care would be of a standard consistent with that practised at the Middlesex and that admission into the ward would not be a problem.

The Team only becomes involved if the person is unable to attend the clinic or there are specific needs relating to symptom control or issues of death and dying. Where there is shared care with clinic staff, the early misunderstandings over interdisciplinary boundaries seem to have been effectively overcome by having case conferences for the more complex problems. Where Team involvement has restored a person's health sufficiently for him or her to return to the out-patients department, the willingness of the Team to refer back has alleviated some anxieties over 'ownership', but, in all quarters, this concern will only evaporate completely with time.

Issues of geography

Over 80 per cent of the clients attending James Pringle House are not resident within Bloomsbury Health District. While the majority come from the metropolis, a significant proportion are scattered through the Home Counties or even further afield. It was therefore important to be aware of the scatter of our potential clients and, at an early stage, establish lines of communication, training and facilitation to enable appropriate referral on to more local agencies. The map (Fig. 7) shows the 60 patients cared for during one year. There have only been 10 resident within Bloomsbury; the majority lie within our arbitrary boundary of one hour's travelling time. A rational use of community resource would incorporate referral between the teams from a number of hospitals. Unfortunately, this is as yet very limited, and is likely to be slow as the territorial issues that are apparently a threat are not geographical.

Figure 7 Geographical location of patients cared for by the BCCT

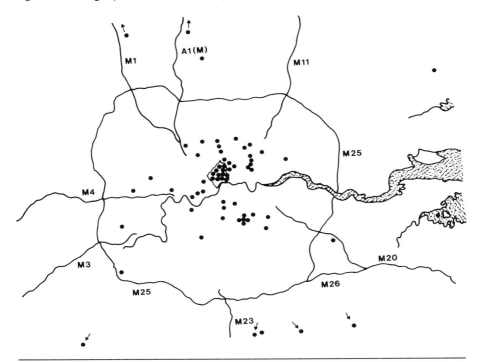

Currently, the levels of service provided are as follows:

- *Levels of care within one hour's travelling time.* This service is designed to complement existing facilities comprehensively and includes:
    — advice on symptom control, diagnosis and nursing.
    — practical back-up for other professionals.
    — 24-hour, 7-day-a-week cover.
    — appropriate support and counselling for patients, relatives and other carers.
    — bereavement follow-up.

The one-hour 'boundary' may well shrink as the patient load increases. At the moment the Team is committed to remaining small and to facilitating a high level of competence within all community and hospice services.

- *Levels of care outside primary geographical area.* This in essence is a secondary backup service:
    — networking
    — facilitation   according to local service provision
    — referral-on
    — advice to advisers
    — admission facilities   via on-call and telephone
    — overview of care

Currently we are examining the geographical distribution of all people with HIV infection attending James Pringle House to describe the scatter of this population so that we can make some estimate of projected needs in the future. This will assist in the liaison with certain key districts or existing continuing care facilities, with other HIV-dedicated services and with the hospice movement in general.

While the initial response of the hospice movement to the problem of terminal care and AIDS was cool, there is now, fortunately, a clearer understanding of needs. In co-operation with Help the Hospices, plans are being made to provide formal training and linking between AIDS services and those caring for people with other terminal conditions.

General practitioners and primary health care teams

This leads on to the other potential difficulty – namely, the apparent resistance of some people with AIDS to the involvement of general practitioners in their management. This has been principally in response to the spectre of confidentiality being breached within the surgery by, say, receptionists, and the concern that attitudes may be unhelpful or skills may be missing from many general practices.

Under the supervision of a local GP and Senior Health Adviser, this issue was clarified at JPH by questioning a group of people with AIDS. Those who had availed themselves of primary health care facilities were by and large satisfied, impressed and very well served. The Team's experience has been very much in keeping with this.

We have found formalised training sessions for general practitioners to have been an abject failure, as yet another evening meeting or study day in an already busy schedule seems to have too low a priority. We have therefore begun to pursue alternative means of educating primary carers following discussions with the local Family Practitioner Committee. These include:

- speaking to group practices on their own territory.
- using individual cases for training and teaching based around shared care. This has been the most effective means of education.
- contributing regularly to the FPC circulars by producing a bi-monthly newsletter in a broadsheet format, the idea being to maintain levels of awareness in a palatable and digestible way.
- The planned publication of leaflets covering specific issues and a modular manual on community care in HIV and AIDS (*see below*).

It was very much the view of the FPC that these training inputs should be for the whole primary team with an emphasis on multi-disciplinary care.

Shared Care Cards

Initiated by a local GP in conjunction with voluntary agencies, this collaborative venture (*see* Fig. 8) was designed principally to overcome the problems of confidentiality, thereby making more patients willing to use primary health care facilities. The additional benefit of client-carried notes is that relevant clinical information and results are available to the whole spectrum of health care professionals involved at any one time, with significant improvements in communication and liaison. The card provides space for medication, clinical notes, results, personal details and appropriate contact addresses for agencies in the statutory and voluntary sector.

These notes are not seen as rendering hospital or GP notes obsolete, but they do mean that specific references to HIV infection need not appear in these relatively public documents.

Nursing

The level of interest and expertise varies enormously both within and between districts. The most pressing issue with respect to community nurses is the lack of training on the basic issues around AIDS and infection control, even within the inner London districts. Aside from training and facilitation of district nurses in primary health care centres, members of the Team are making regular contributions to several nursing courses on AIDS in the London regions and at the Royal College of Nursing. We have also contributed to a wide spectrum of meetings on AIDS and terminal care.

Social services

The problems of housing and service provision within inner city authorities are by no means unique to AIDS and they are best debated elsewhere. Suffice it to say that there is an acute and escalating need for all forms of accommodation, but particularly for places where there is some degree of

Figure 8 Shared Care Cards

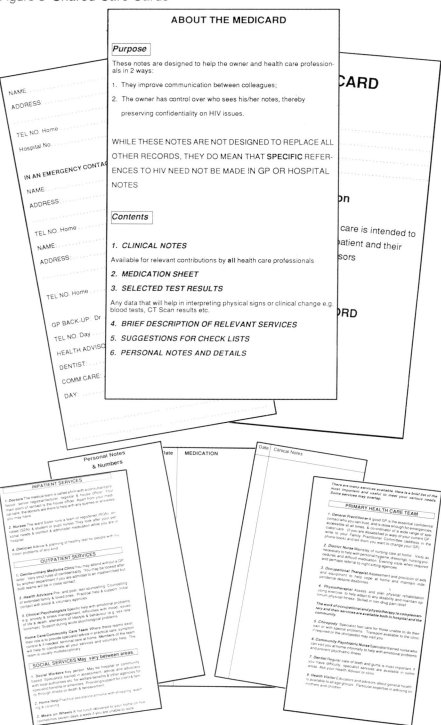

support or supervision for those with visual, neurological or intellectual difficulties. The specific needs of drug users are not being addressed at all at present.

There has been a major positive response for guidance from the local authorities that overlap Bloomsbury, and hopefully the series of teaching seminars done by the Team on the broad issues around AIDS will bear fruit.

Literature

The need for accurate and appropriate literature for patients, carers and professionals is increasingly evident, especially in the areas of loss – ranging from physical loss, such as eyesight and mobility or mental function, through to bereavement. Having established a base of experience, the Team plans to make some contribution to this area in the next year.

The next main project is the development of a modular manual – *The Bloomsbury Manual of Community Care in HIV and AIDS* – covering all issues that health care professionals are likely to encounter in the community in relation to HIV and AIDS. While the bulk of the writing is being done by appropriate members of the Team, we will also be drawing on the enormous depth of expertise within Bloomsbury to provide a comprehensive manual.

The objectives of using a modular ring binder system are that key sections can be updated and that individuals can produce personalised documents. We anticipate that this will be available in the middle of 1989.

The spectrum of informal care structures

The definition or use of the term 'family' is, in a sense, difficult as we all have preconceptions. Our current experience is that many individuals with HIV-related disease, while having partners and/or many friends, frequently have schisms with, for example, their blood relatives or tensions between family and partners or other carers. Consequently, for many the assumption that there is a baseline of primary care which will come from the 'family' is not realistic. However, there is an overwhelming response, particularly within the gay community, to the needs of individuals with AIDS such that extended care structures, while being *ad hoc*, are often very effective. One must, however, be mindful that this type of community support may be a luxury not available in low-incidence areas. In many circumstances, the creation of support around an individual requires considerable flexibility and the need to marshal resources in an appropriate way. For example, adequate provision of cover around the clock for a person dying at home alone is likely to consume in excess of 12 volunteers.

Links with the voluntary sector

To have workable relationships with people in the voluntary sector has really been dependent upon close personal contact over cases. In addition, key people have been identified within relevant organisations, and they are met with regularly in a very informal way for update and feedback. This has led to good co-operation.

Contact has also been made with three Community Health Councils (CHCs), particularly with respect to feedback on hospital services. In addition, the Team is providing desk-top publishing facilities for a quarterly newsletter produced by a CHC and a voluntary agency, which has been well received. Using the newsletter format, we hope to promote more communication and debate on issues surrounding the care of people with AIDS, especially the needs of the ethnic minorities and specific issues such as housing and legal problems. This is turning out to be a very successful venture.

It is particularly in this area that close linking with the voluntary sector – and especially agencies such as Frontliners, Body Positive and the Terrence Higgins Trust – has been valuable. The establishment of the new trust ACET (AIDS, Care, Education & Training), with a specific brief for home and continuing care, is expected to provide a significant additional resource, assuming things proceed effectively.

Bereavement

We do not have enough experience so far to make anything other than broad statements in this area. The Team provides follow-up on all people close to someone's death to enable us to pick up on potential problems with complicated grief. These people are then referred on to an appropriate agency should the need arise.

Two clear issues around AIDS do increase the likelihood of problems in these early years. Social stigma still means that the true diagnosis is usually only known to close family. For many, the inability to share 'what really went on' will obstruct normal grief. Connected with this, partners or lovers may be fearful that the diagnosis will lead to speculations about their possible drug use or lifestyle. In addition, there is still no clear status of bereavement available to the partner of a gay man. Finally, many people are experiencing multiple bereavements as the virus has manifested itself in the 'closed' sub-cultures. The tendency for many to sublimate their grief in voluntary work must be looked at very carefully as it is endemic, not least because the early political and practical work of the early 1980s was done by those who had been affected first hand.

The Team

Obviously it is difficult to be objective about a team in which one author was the first member, particularly as we are still at an early stage. Nevertheless, one or two general points are worth making.

Team dynamics

The appointment of a small team comprising professionals accredited with experience and leadership within their own spheres could have been a formula for fireworks. Instead, it has been crucial to the survival of the group. For example, the pressures to perform and succeed, while to some extent internally generated, have been profound. It is difficult to imagine how people without maturity and insight would have managed without experiencing significant personal problems. This is an important take-home message for those wishing to initiate work in this area.

There have been the inevitable tensions and confusions as our role has evolved – both as 'the Team' in relating to other 'teams', and as individual professionals relating within 'the Team' – but these have been trivial. Each individual is theoretically responsible to managers in his/her individual speciality, yet also has responsibilities within the Team. Potential confusion over line management has been overcome with a staunch defence of consensus, and by the Team visibly identifying with any member in difficulty. The overwhelming commitment of every member to have this venture succeed has meant that issues have been addressed and resolved as soon as conflict has arisen. The particular pressures of work dealing with death and dying have been heightened by the age group involved, the complexity of the disease, the political profile, time pressure and the deluge of patients. The gestation and development that one would ordinarily have expected to take two years were compressed into about six months without any loss of staff.

Team building
The weekly business meeting has allowed a regular forum for discussion and has been the fulcrum of Team life; patient sharing has meant that members have functioned in a transdisciplinary way. This has allowed everyone to gain maximum experience, and has also meant that the risk of clinical or emotional isolation has been minimised. The disadvantage is that there may be unequal role-sharing or loss of professional identity, particularly as many patients are inclined to attach different significance to a visit from the nurse, social worker or doctor. It is most important within the process of team building to affirm role and to educate those outside that each member represents the corporation.

Support
The definitions of 'support' and 'counselling' are apt to be confused, particularly when discussing Team life. The commitment to each other and concern for mutual welfare, together with our corporate experience as team members, have meant that there has been substantial support within the Team, particularly for members who have had hostility from other agencies, but this in itself is not sufficient. It was realised early on that every member might need independent help, and so all are expected to use counsellors of their own choice during Team time, and this is paid for from the budget if they wish. There have also been several days or half days set aside to look at key issues. These have served to crystallise areas of weakness and strength, and have been most valuable.

It is easy to see how people working alone in this field are at major risk of burn-out. It seems clear that only a limited number of areas in the UK will need specialised teams, yet most areas will need some expansion of their current continuing care services, by one or more workers. We would emphasise the need for these initiatives to be firmly supported and, where possible, attached to established projects from which the workers can gain some identity.

Table 4 **Bloomsbury Community Care Team summary of workload, December 1987–January 1989**

Total no. of patients seen	64 (62 male, 2 female) (63 AIDS, 1 HIV+ve)
Risk factor	59 homosexual 2 injecting drug use 2 bisexual 1 heterosexual
Average no. in Team's care at any one time	20
Source of referral	30 Clinic 24 Hospital 2 GP 8 Other
GP/PHCT involvement	37
Mean time with Team until death	8 weeks
Respite care	9 admitted for respite care (7 to Mildmay); maximum 6 weeks' respite care
No. of patients referred on	8
No. of deaths	38
Place of death	20 Home 9 Hospice 9 Hospital
Bereavement follow-up	25 relatives

Areas for expansion

Clinical The Team still picks up on many people who have no general practitioner, and the therapeutic/palliative boundaries are very variable. Hence the amount of specialist nursing and, in particular, medical input and expertise has been greater than might have been suggested by the experience with cancer. Coupled with the increasing requests for education and the need for research, there is an urgent need for additional medical sessions. The Team is likely to expand by one person at least.

Other disciplines Occupational therapy is the major discipline that should have some clearer Team representation. Most patients wish to maintain their independence as long as possible, and it would appear that an increasing number are troubled with neurological deficit. A specialist post has been created to combine ward and community work, and this person will have a flexible number of sessions with BCCT. A similar arrangement has been formulated with dietetics, and this extension of the service is working well. The needs for physiotherapy as yet seem adequately covered using existing provisions.

Conclusions

This venture is still in its infancy. On the positive side, it seems to be contributing significantly to the spectrum of care needs expressed by those with AIDS. However, objective evaluation will not really be available for another 12 months.

Table 4 shows a summary of the workload to date. In less than one year, the client capacity has reached that of an established cancer team. While this reflects the size of this clinical problem in central London, the success so far is more likely to be a synthesis of the skills of those within the Team, coupled with the willingness of other professionals to use the service.

On the negative side, education of and devolution to other services are lagging behind needs. How much of this is due to the existence of the Team is difficult to know. Suffice it to say, the stresses of providing a service and trying to make things happen, as opposed to doing them, is considerable. No planner should consider such services without exploring the potential of expanding existing resources and considering the calibre and structure of any initiative that they may need.

References

Carne, C. A., Weller, I. V. D., Johnson, A. M. *et al.* (1987) Prevalence of antibodies to human immunodeficiency virus, gonorrhoea rates and changing sexual behaviour in homosexual men in London. *Lancet* (i), 656–8.

Des Jarlais, D. C. and Friedman, S. R. (1987) HIV infection among intravenous drug users: epidemiology and risk reduction. *AIDS* 1, 67–76.

Ferlie, E. and Pettigrew, A. (1988) *The Management of Change in Bloomsbury DHA: AIDS and acute sector strategy.* Centre for Corporate Strategy and Change, University of Warwick.

Hart, G. J., Carvell, A., Johnson, A. M. *et al.* (1988) Needle-exchange – a public health response to HIV infection amongst injecting drug users. Paper presented at Society for Social Medicine conference, Newcastle.

Hart, G. J., Sonnex, C., Petherick, A. *et al.* (1989) Risk behaviours for HIV infection amongst injecting intravenous drug users attending a drug dependency clinic. *British Medical Journal* (in press).

Robertson, J. R., Bucknall, A. B. V., Welsby, P. D. *et al.* (1986) Epidemic of AIDS-related virus' (HTLV-III/LAV) infection among intravenous drug abusers. *British Medical Journal* 292, 527–9.

Shilts, R. (1988) *And the Band Played On.* London, Penguin.

HIV Infection and AIDS in Lothian

Dr Alison M. Richardson and Dr Philip A. Gaskell

Lothian Region

Lothian Region is a local authority area of approximately 700 square miles and consists of the four districts of Mid, East and West Lothian and Edinburgh City. Each district has its own distinctive character, the three surrounding Edinburgh maintain agricultural land, while West and Mid Lothian also having areas of mineral and coal deposits. The population statistics are shown in Table 5.

Edinburgh is the administrative capital of Scotland and is a major cultural, educational, legal, financial and tourist centre. Service industries predominate, and there has been a decline in manufacturing employment. As of August 1988, unemployment in Edinburgh stood at 10.2 per cent over all, although the rate for males was 12.8 per cent.

Health services

Lothian Health Board has seven health service units, two hospital based and the others service or geographically organised. There are a total of 35 hospitals and 8,458 in-patient beds.

The Royal Infirmary and the Western General Hospital in Edinburgh are the major general hospitals providing a full range of acute services. These, and other hospitals in the area, are teaching hospitals and also provide specialist services for neighbouring health boards. For example, the Infectious Diseases Unit, based at the City Hospital, gave an early response to the problems associated with HIV-related disease and remains an important research centre with vital contacts in the community.

Table 5 **Population of the Lothian Region by district (1988)**

East Lothian	81,855
Mid Lothian	81,440
West Lothian	141,684
Edinburgh City	438,721
Total	743,700

Primary care services

There are 510 general practitioners working in 150 practices. Fifty of these have trainee assistants; in addition undergraduates are taught by attachment to local practices for four weeks. There are 14 health centres, and, during the last five years, 13 new group practice premises have been built using the NHS Cost Rent Scheme. The views of GPs are represented to the Lothian Health Board by an elected General Practitioner Subcommittee of the Area Medical Committee.

The University of Edinburgh Department of General Practice acts as a focus for GP teaching and research in the area. The quality, quantity and originality of recent GP research on drug misuse and HIV infection have been important.

Existing Links

Formal links exist between the Health Board and local authorities in the form of the Joint Health Liaison Committee. There is already co-operation in the areas of personal social services, housing and education. In addition, Joint Committees were established in response to the SHAPE (Scottish Health Authorities' Priorities for the Eighties) Report in 1985. These will report on needs and co-ordinate voluntary, health board and social work activity in the spheres of mental illness, mental handicap, the elderly and the young disabled.

The prevalence of HIV infection

As elsewhere, the prevalence of HIV infection within Lothian is unknown. Estimated figures are provided through the Communicable Diseases (Scotland) Unit which monitors the antibody-positive reports from the Scottish Health Service laboratories. While these figures may be inflated by duplicate tests on the same patient in different settings, the total is certain to be a considerable underestimate of the numbers of infected individuals within Lothian. Table 6 shows the cumulative totals of HIV-positive results and people with AIDS in Scotland. Table 7 gives a breakdown by transmission category.

Of all Scottish HIV antibody-positive reports, 60 per cent are from the Edinburgh area, with a further 22 per cent reported from Glasgow. The most salient feature of HIV infection in Lothian is illustrated by the fact that injecting drug users constitute at least 54 per cent of those infected in the area. *It is now estimated that, in the City of Edinburgh, 1 per cent of males between the ages of 15 and 45 are infected* (Lothian Health Board, 1988).

By the end of October 1988, 68 cases of AIDS had been reported to the Communicable Diseases (Scotland) Unit, 32 of whom had died. Estimates given in the Tayler Report (1987) predicted that there would be a

Table 6 Cumulative totals of HIV antibody-positive reports and people with AIDS in Scotland to 30 September 1988

	HIV antibody-positive reports	*People with AIDS*
Male	1031	59
Female	418	8
Not stated	96	–
Total	1545	67

From data made available by the Communicable Diseases (Scotland) Unit

cumulative total of 130–227 cases of AIDS in Scotland by 1991 with a doubling time of 12 months, with the vast majority of cases expected in Lothian. Given that between 50 and 60 per cent of current cases are young heterosexuals, the potential for heterosexual transmission is probably greater in Lothian than anywhere else in the UK.

It has been difficult to communicate the urgency of the problem when, so far, there have been relatively few deaths, but it is clear that Lothian will soon have to contend with a very large number of people becoming ill and dying.

The majority of those identified in Lothian as HIV positive or as having AIDS are local residents, but some attend clinics from other areas of Scotland, particularly the adjacent regions of Fife and the Borders. Some have also returned to Edinburgh from other areas of the country in order to be with their families before death.

Initial impact

AIDS initially became a local issue when it was discovered that Lothian had an unaccountably high incidence of HIV infection in drug users. The Edinburgh Drug Addiction Study had been set up in 1984, based in one general practice whose patients included a large number of drug users. In 1985, it was found, from stored serum, that 51 per cent of the study group were HIV infected and had become so between 1983 and 1985 (Robertson *et al.*, 1986). Other surveys provided similar results (e.g. Peutherer *et al.*, 1985; Brettle *et al.*, 1987). All this suggested a much higher rate of infection among injecting drug users than had been reported in any other part of the UK and, indeed, higher than in many parts of Europe and the United States.

These findings were raised by the media as a moral and a public health issue. For the statutory agencies, there was clearly an urgent need to provide services for those with HIV infection and AIDS. However, for those

Table 7 Percentage distribution by transmission category of HIV-positive reports in Scotland to 30 September 1988

	Male	Female	Not stated	Total
Homosexual/ bisexual contact	23.6	–	–	15.4
Injecting drug use	52.5	66.7	26.1	54.7
Recipient of blood/ blood products	7.9	1.0	1.0	5.5
Heterosexual contact	3.0	12.9	1.0	5.6
Child	1.7	6.0	30.2	4.7
Others/unknown	11.3	13.4	41.7	14.1

From data made available by the Communicable Diseases (Scotland) Unit

infected in 1983 and 1984, prevention was too late, and, to a large extent, the need to react to an existing problem has dominated the local response.

The City of Edinburgh was remarkable in having virtually no statutory agencies dealing with drug problems. As a result, the burden of care had fallen largely on voluntary agencies. Treatment of drug problems in Lothian has therefore become a dominant issue in the prevention and provision of treatment for HIV and AIDS.

The McClelland Committee was constituted by the Scottish Home and Health Department (SHHD) in February 1986, and its final report *HIV in Scotland* (1986) was undoubtedly important in initiating a more coherent response from both hospital and community services. In particular, the report tackled the difficult areas of provision of injecting equipment and of substitute prescribing, and made the important statement that

> *authorities should be reminded that threat to life of the spread of HIV infection is greater than that of drug misuse. On balance, the prevention of spread should take priority over any perceived risk of increased drug misuse.*

The McClelland Committee was remarkable for the fact that it made its report in the space of only five months, an indication of the members' perception of the urgency of the problem.

Before this report had been published, a counselling and screening clinic had been set up at the City Hospital's Infectious Diseases Unit, largely through the individual initiative of Dr Ray Brettle who campaigned from an early stage for appropriate drug services. He initiated substitute prescribing for both HIV-infected and uninfected drug users who attended for screening and medical advice. Despite many initial problems, this service provided the impetus for the first statutory responses to the drug problems in Lothian, and added to an increasing awareness among general practitioners and other community services that the problem could no longer be ignored.

At the same time, information about the risk of HIV infection was provided by local and national media, and this was associated with a large increase in the number of patients seen at the Department of Genito-urinary Medicine (GUM) at the Royal Infirmary in Edinburgh. This hospital department and the City Hospital's Infectious Diseases Unit have continued to be the focus of treatment services for HIV and AIDS. The Infectious Diseases Unit is seen to be the service for potentially infected drug users, while the GUM clinic has identified the majority of homosexual men found to be infected. These differences were not planned and they are disappearing as infected people choose which clinic they attend. The general public approach both clinics for HIV testing, as do those who have been at risk through injecting drugs or engaging in possible high-risk behaviour. As the epidemic progresses, each clinic will probably need to gain more expertise in areas with which they are less familiar: the detection and treatment of other sexually transmitted diseases by the City Hospital and the management of drug users by the GUM clinic.

There have been individual initiatives within the community, too. Dr Roy Robertson and Dr Kennedy Roberts of the Edinburgh Drug Addiction Study, who are general practitioners in an area of Edinburgh where there is a high rate of both drug misuse and HIV infection, also stand out as those who, at an early stage, both recognised the extent of the problem and responded to it in the community. Continuing collaboration between the City Hospital and this general practice is important in developing expertise in and research into HIV infection and AIDS within Lothian and in providing care for infected people.

Organisational responses

A variety of intra- and inter-agency groups and committees have been set up in response to the AIDS problem in Lothian and, although in a continuing state of development, both statutory and non-statutory bodies are represented directly or indirectly. The major committees which have come into existence in response to the problem are shown in Table 8.

Table 8 Organisational response to HIV and AIDS in Lothian (not an exhaustive list)

- *The Lothian AIDS Advisory Group* which operates as a source of medical advice on technical and patient-related aspects of AIDS.

- *The AIDS Co-ordinating Group* whose remit is to implement the Health Board's agreed plans for the AIDS services.

- *The AIDS Regional Group* at which regional council, social work, Health Board and voluntary group representatives meet to advise on the establishment and co-ordination of services for HIV and AIDS.

- *The AIDS Strategic Planning Group* involving those employed by the Health Board specifically for AIDS services, who are developing a strategy for prevention and treatment services.

- *The General Practitioner Group,* formed to translate local GP expertise into co-ordinated encouragement, support, education and action.

- *The AIDS Resource Group,* bringing together professionals from a variety of disciplines who are willing to give input to agencies who request information about HIV and AIDS.

- *The AIDS Research Co-ordination Group* comprising clinical, university and other staff working in the area either directly or peripherally.

As a direct result of the McClelland Report, Lothian Health Board now employ an AIDS co-ordinator (a community medicine specialist), a health promotion officer, an administrator and a community outreach worker who, together, constitute the 'AIDS team'. Also as a result of this report, other personnel were taken on by the Board specifically to work with those who are HIV infected.

The agencies which have had most impact within the non-statutory sector are Scottish AIDS Monitor (SAM) and the drug projects. SAM is a voluntary organisation which provides a variety of services for those who are infected with HIV; its equivalent in England is the Terrence Higgins Trust. The drug projects have a vital role to play in the Lothian region because of the dearth of statutory services. Links between drug services are provided by an Edinburgh Drugs Action Group.

There has also been a proliferation of groups at both local and regional levels. The local groups, based in the communities with large numbers of drug users, serve to inform, educate and stimulate individual initiatives, and to provide support for those working with drug users. In general, the health, social and voluntary services are well represented as, increasingly, are representatives of the communities.

Until comparatively recently, there was little involvement from GPs, perhaps because only a few practices provided most of the health care to drug users and other GPs had not yet felt the impact of the HIV problem. There is sometimes a reluctance among infected members of the gay and drug-using communities to involve their GPs, preferring to have their health care needs met by the hospital services. The General Practitioner Group, formed in January 1988, is therefore an important development in terms of community care.

Funding and resources

Again, following the McClelland Report, the Health Board identified separate funding for AIDS services. Some of this has been provided from within existing budgets, but there has also been direct additional funding for different projects from the SHHD. Voluntary drug groups and SAM receive such funding.

Services are gradually being developed which are specifically dedicated towards the AIDS problem. The counselling clinic was the first of these, funded initially from the Scottish Office as a research programme, and subsequently by the Health Board. Since then, in addition to funding for the AIDS team, two clinical psychology posts and a variety of nursing, secretarial and clerical posts have been established by the Health Board at the Royal Infirmary and the City Hospital.

Further funding from the Scottish Office is aimed at providing a whole range of medical, nursing and ancillary services which will be gradually integrated into the existing Infectious Diseases Unit at the City Hospital. In May 1988, the SHHD agreed to fund the capital and revenue costs for a 15-bed AIDS unit at the City Hospital as an integrated part of the Infectious Diseases Department. It was originally scheduled for completion in 1990, but now seems unlikely to be ready until the following year.

Prevention and health promotion

Preventive activities take place on two different levels. The Scottish Health Education Group (SHEG) is broadly responsible for health education in the same way that HEA is in England. SHEG has been involved in providing a programme of courses and workshops for nurse educators in Scotland and in developing an AIDS counselling and resources pack. There are also a variety of Health Board, regional and social service initiatives aimed at the prevention of spread, health and safety and health promotion. Specific workshops have been organised for those working directly and indirectly with HIV-infected people, and a concerted public education campaign about safer sex has been planned to begin on Valentine's Day 1989.

Various organisations have put forward proposals for health education. It is unfortunate that these are not always well co-ordinated and that different agencies appear to be duplicating effort.

The AIDS Resource Group was convened by the Health Board AIDS co-ordinator in early 1987. This brought together professionals from health, social work and education with representatives of Lothian Region and Edinburgh District Councils. In its first year of operation, this group responded to requests from a variety of agencies seeking information about HIV/AIDS, most requests concerning health and safety. A recent review has established the need for the group to take the initiative and to concentrate more on attitudes and behaviour.

There have been numerous initiatives through trade unions, trade associations and other professional bodies who have taken AIDS education to their members. The AIDS Resource Group offers help with such projects. Community (previously 'adult' or 'further') education provides education for voluntary youth workers, and this has proved to be an effective means of reaching young people.

A National AIDS Line, a local SAM phoneline which operates in the evening, and a phoneline at the counselling clinic at the City Hospital are all used by the general public as well as by those who are directly affected by the problems of HIV. The number of calls – particularly from the 'worried well' – varies enormously, largely depending on media campaigns.

Three needle exchanges were set up in Scotland in April 1987, and of these the one in Edinburgh has been most successful, perhaps largely because of the lack of opposition in the local community and the relative anonymity of its location. The relative success of the Edinburgh exchange cannot, however, hide its inadequacies in comparison with similar projects south of the border. This does not reflect on those actually running the project, who have devoted considerable time and expertise to trying to make it a success. Rather, restrictions imposed in Scotland (for example, because of the law) have made it difficult to expand the exchange to a level where it can contact more than a fraction of the drug-using population. This is regarded as a serious shortcoming in Lothian where needle sharing has clearly contributed to the high level of infection. It is notable that the proposal of a new needle exchange in a different area of the city has been given considerable support from local people after a spate of 'needlestick' injuries in children who came across used needles in a local park. Unfortunately, six months later, the Scottish Office had still not given permission for this exchange to go ahead.

The sale of injecting equipment from pharmacies has also recently been approved by SHHD, and one of the local drug agencies also provides clean equipment for injecting drug users.

A Community Drugs Problem Service (CDPS) has been started by Lothian Health Board, as much in response to the problem of HIV infection as to drug misuse. This new service, which consists, so far, of a consultant psychiatrist and two community psychiatric nurses, is a particularly important development since it is Lothian's first local specialist health service initiative towards managing the drugs problem. It is regarded as long overdue by most agencies. The service is described in detail in a later section.

Service provision

The hospitals
Services for HIV-infected people and AIDS patients are provided by three separate hospital services.

Haemophiliacs
The number of HIV-positive haemophiliacs in Lothian is small in comparison with some other areas of the country. They are cared for separately from the other AIDS services by the Haematology Department of the Royal Infirmary. The team consists of service and research doctors, specialist haemophilia nurses and social workers, with regular input from a clinical psychologist and a psychiatrist. Extra finance has added a half-time medical associate and a half-time social worker in response to the HIV dimension. Both out-patient and in-patient treatment are carried out by the same staff within a general medical ward.

City Hospital: Infectious Diseases Unit
The majority of infected drug users are treated at the City Hospital Infectious Diseases Unit in Edinburgh. This unit is, to date, the focus for screening, counselling and in-patient treatment. Anyone who wishes to have an HIV antibody test may approach this service confidentially and will be counselled prior to having the test carried out. Those who are found to be HIV positive are invited to attend the medical clinic, where their medical status is regularly monitored every three months. Currently, 88 per cent of those attending this clinic were infected directly through injecting drug use or through sexual contact with a drug user. Those who have medical problems requiring in-patient treatment are admitted to one of the general infectious diseases wards. There is no segregation of HIV-positive or AIDS patients. Infected children are also seen at this clinic and at the Royal Hospital for Sick Children.

Royal Infirmary of Edinburgh: Department of Genito-urinary Medicine
This department also looks after a number of infected and 'at risk' individuals. The majority of such patients are homosexual men, but the department also treats a significant number of current and former drug

users, and it is frequently approached by people who feel that they are at risk through heterosexual intercourse.

The philosophy of this department differs from that of the City Hospital in that there is greater emphasis on the need for screening for sexually transmitted diseases because of the different nature of many of the presentations. Patients are therefore more likely to be seen by a doctor than a counsellor on their first visit, and almost all patients who attend asking for an 'AIDS test' will be fully screened for sexually transmitted diseases. Patients are largely treated on an out-patient basis, those requiring in-patient treatment being admitted either to a general medical ward in the Royal Infirmary or to the City Hospital.

Day and terminal care
Currently, there is no separate provision for either day care or terminal care within Lothian Region, although terminal care is provided at the City Hospital Infectious Diseases Unit. There has been lengthy discussion among a variety of agencies about these aspects of care.

Under consideration at present is a proposal for an AIDS resource centre. There are premises available, but funding for both capital and revenue expenditure is still being sought. It would provide a walk-in day centre for infected people and provide a community base from which a variety of statutory and non-statutory agencies could operate.

The Tayler Report (1987) recommended that a 15-bed hospice should be established in Edinburgh 'as soon as possible'. However, a joint council and voluntary group plan to set up such a hospice in West Lothian foundered, partly because of the unsuitability of the proposed premises but also under the heavy weight of local opposition. The media attention which this Torphichen project received was unhelpful in that it generated considerable heat between the proposers and the local community. There were many objections on the grounds that the hospice would be too far from the patients' own communities and ill served by public transport, but these considerations were largely left to one side and reporting tended to reflect the anti-AIDS nature of the argument. Both Lothian Region and the Milestone Trust are continuing to pursue the need for hospice care in Lothian, and existing hospices are co-operating in the planning of this response.

Testing
There is no clear policy about testing consent procedures in Lothian. In particular, the laboratories and the Health Board have not decided to follow the policy of informed consent of patients with their written permission. There have consequently been numerous cases in which informed consent was not obtained, though that does not occur in the units with most experience of HIV disease.

Within the Infectious Diseases Unit and the GUM clinic, the two departments most concerned with the problem, there are clear policies about testing and consent, but it is unfortunately true that these policies differ to some degree. At the Infectious Diseases Unit, no one is tested without counselling, and screening for sexually transmitted disease is not necessarily carried out. At the GUM clinic, on the other hand, the majority are screened for sexually transmitted diseases in the first instance.

Both departments have firm guidelines about confidentiality so that patients can be tested for HIV without their GPs' knowledge. In both clinics, self-referrals are common, and it is known that many give false names and addresses in order to ensure that they cannot be identified. If patients are found to be antibody-positive, strenuous attempts are made to persuade them to inform their GPs and, if they are unwilling to do so, to change to a GP in whom they would feel able to confide. Only a very small minority of patients refuse to do so, though there is often initial resistance.

Social Work Department

Since 1986, the Social Work Department has been providing foster care and nursery places for children born to HIV-positive women. The majority of work for these services was undertaken using existing resources, although extra staff were appointed during 1987 and 1988. These include AIDS advisers, a training officer and support workers within the supported-accommodation team, and recently, provision has been made for family finders for children, hospital social workers and social workers specifically employed to work with drug users.

Staff training

Specific staff training programmes were set up by the Social Work Department for their staff, particularly social workers, home-helps and nursery staff. Potential foster parents also receive training.

Within the Health Board, staff training occurs on a more haphazard basis, with input from the AIDS team but, in many cases, provided at a local hospital level. There are immediate plans for training programmes at the City Hospital, where a questionnaire has assessed the knowledge, attitudes and behaviour of staff with regard to HIV infection.

However, such training often appears to be reacting to needs rather than taking the lead. It should be emphasised that the perceived need lies more with those who are not in frequent contact with patients than with those who work directly with them. Concern is more often expressed about the presence of drug users than of those people with HIV infection. The need for training is most apparent in hospitals which have so far had little direct experience of caring for HIV-positive patients; here, such patients continue to complain that they are treated insensitively, being required to use their own cutlery and plates, asked to use separate toilet facilities and their visitors being advised to put on gowns. Further training of hospital staff is clearly of major importance, but there often appears to be a measure of complacency and sometimes even hostility from those whose major concern is with patients with other illnesses. If people with AIDS are perceived as receiving resources denied to other patients, this attitude is perhaps understandable in the present NHS climate.

Information and research

Information is held by each clinic about the numbers who attend for testing and seropositivity rates. All this information is confidential and is not usually shared between agencies. Generally, confidentiality is paramount although this may occasionally interfere with the useful transfer of information.

The majority of information at the City Hospital is currently collected through research studies being carried out by staff there. This information is concerned with AIDS and HIV prevalence and clinical and laboratory indicators of the progress of the disease and its response to treatment. Information has not been collected about workload, costings, etc., although the requirements of the AIDS Control Act now ensure that more information is collated.

At present, laboratories report the number of positive tests that they process, giving additional information where that is available. They are dependent on information given to them which is often incomplete, and there is little information on those tested and found negative. A new computer-based recording system has been recently introduced into all Scottish laboratories which should enable better information to be collected.

There are a number of research studies in progress, mainly locally based. These include:
- A study of infected and uninfected haemophiliacs, looking at clinical and laboratory measures of their medical status.
- The effect of pregnancy on HIV infection.
- The natural history of perinatally acquired HIV infection.
- The natural history of HIV infection in injecting drug users.
- A neurophysiological and neuropsychological study of early HIV infection.
- A study of heterosexual transmission of HIV.
- The Edinburgh Drug Addiction Study which has been following up 201 injecting drug users since 1984.

The above projects all involve health service staff and are carried out through clinics. Some are part of national studies, while others are locally based. There are also a variety of research studies which have emanated from the University of Edinburgh. These include specialised scientific projects into HIV itself and on the diagnosis of pneumocystis carinii, as well as behavioural and psychosocial studies, both within 'risk groups' and in the wider community. There is a very real concern among some workers that the infected population is being over researched, and that efforts should be made to ensure that these research activities do not interfere with the care and treatment of individuals.

Local issues

Edinburgh has been called 'the AIDS Capital of the North' due to the large number of injecting drug users within the city who are infected with HIV. By October 1985, when this was discovered, it was estimated that 40 per cent had been infected, compared with a probable 4 per cent in the West of Scotland and 33 per cent in Tayside (Tayler Report, 1987).

Within Lothian, it is therefore difficult to differentiate between the issues surrounding drug misuse and those of HIV infection and AIDS. It is, of course, important to remember that there are almost as many people infected in Lothian who are *not and never have been* injecting drug users. Of those who were infected through needle sharing, a large percentage are now abstaining from intravenous use, and many are not using illicit drugs at all. The fact that the following sections deal primarily with drug issues should not, therefore, be seen as representing the whole picture of HIV infection in Lothian Region. However, because of the nature of the infected population in Lothian, there is a very real concern that Edinburgh will experience the first wave of infection within the heterosexual, non-drug-using population in the UK.

Drug problems

To understand the particular difficulties experienced in Lothian, a number of important factors must be taken into account, although it remains uncertain to what extent these were influential in the spread of HIV in Edinburgh. The Lothian Drug Squad estimate that, throughout the 1970s, there were perhaps 40–50 heroin users in Lothian. However, in the early 1980s, there was a rapid increase, mainly centred on four council housing schemes in Edinburgh. Supplies of heroin were plentiful, but needles and syringes were scarce. It is generally accepted, though unproven, that, in their management of drug problems and particularly in their dealing with the availability of equipment, the police at that time contributed to an increase in the sharing of needles and syringes. Clean equipment became almost impossible to buy after 1982 when one surgical supplies shop stopped providing it. Thus, the prevailing drug culture, with an emphasis on injection rather than inhalation, played a large part in the spread of HIV among this population (Robertson, Skidmore & Roberts, 1988a).

The Report by the Advisory Council on the Misuse of Drugs (Part 1) (DHSS, 1988) identified some notable features of drug services in Scotland which have also contributed to the situation.

Lack of treatment services

Despite government recommendations to the contrary, expenditure on mental health services in Scotland in general and Lothian in particular has decreased in real terms during the 1980s. Proposals from hospital level to the Health Board and, through it, to the Scottish Office to fund and provide a drugs service were not supported. There was, and continues to be, a dearth of psychiatric input for drug users in Scotland, most notably in Edinburgh. This means that there has been little or no specialist support for those community agencies (usually GPs and voluntary groups) who were prepared to work with the drug-using population. The services which do exist have not always been 'user friendly' or geared towards gradually drawing drug users into contact with helping agencies. A service which initially demands abstinence as a goal is much less likely to attract clients than one which will initially offer support, graduating though maintenance and/or reduction to a similar end. There undoubtedly continues to be profound ambivalence among Scottish psychiatrists regarding their exact role in the management of drug use.

The only available NHS in-patient treatment in Edinburgh was in the acute wards of the main psychiatric hospital, the Royal Edinburgh Hospital, which had been designated as a drug treatment centre. It is fair to point out that the drug users, not seeing themselves as mentally ill, found it extremely difficult to tolerate detoxification in a ward where the majority of patients were being treated for psychotic illnesses. Staff, geared towards the care of psychiatrically disturbed patients, found drug users equally problematic.

Out-patient treatment by the psychiatric services had encompassed maintenance prescribing until the end of the 1970s, but a policy decision to end this was taken at that time because of uncertainty about the role that the service should take. There was concern about the doubtful efficacy of maintenance prescribing. In addition, junior doctors were often put in a difficult position by users demanding drugs, sometimes out of normal hours, and users were thought to be dealing in prescribed drugs on the black market. A very small number of addicts, seen by a forensic psychiatrist, continued to be maintained beyond that time, but few new patients were taken on.

There is major concern about the psychiatric care of those who are affected by HIV disease, including both those who do and those who do not use drugs. Psychiatric help is sought for psychiatric problems but generally not for the 'treatment' of drug misuse. The management of psychiatric illness and dementia in the HIV-infected population is under discussion between primary care, hospital and psychiatric services. Among other matters, the risk of infection seems to be of particular concern to psychiatrists at the Royal Edinburgh Hospital. For their part, the hospital and community services feel that they receive little backup from those who are most experienced in dealing with psychiatric illness. Good will exists in both sectors, and it is hoped that the problems will be resolved. This may take the form of extended psychiatric nursing input to the City Hospital. There is also a proposal that secure accommodation might be provided at the City Hospital and that the Royal Edinburgh Hospital will be able to take those patients who have psychiatric illness and who are not at high risk of transmitting the disease. A consultant in liaison psychiatry (i.e. between hospital and community services) at the City Hospital will shortly be appointed. Without beds or backup, this development is unlikely to solve the problems which are increasingly evident.

Concern about prescribing

There has been considerable reluctance among many doctors to provide a general medical service to drug users. Medical practitioners, as a group, are sharply divided about the wisdom and validity of maintenance prescribing as a means of managing drug use, and the advent of HIV infection has not necessarily persuaded many to view it more positively. In addition, the lack of psychiatric backup may have made GPs more reluctant to take on the task of managing drug users themselves. The role of GPs is explored more fully in a later section.

Equipment provision

Although the McClelland Report (1986) had recommended that clean needles and syringes should be provided, this was not acted on until April 1987, when needle exchange schemes for Edinburgh, Glasgow and Dundee were approved. This delay is just one manifestation of the ambivalence towards this group of patients which has been prevalent within statutory services and at governmental level. The Advisory Council on the Misuse of Drugs (ACMD) Report has pointed out that the pilot needle exchange schemes in Scotland are less 'user friendly' than their counterparts in England. They are medically supervised, are open for only limited periods and may only issue three syringes at any one time. It is hard to find a rationale for the latter, given the limited opening hours of the clinics.

The Scottish Office has recently approved needle supply from pharmacies and, in general, this is welcomed by the statutory agencies. Unfortunately, this has been approved to operate only on a commercial basis and must be unique for being a public health measure for which patients must pay. In September 1988, approval was also given for supply through general practitioners, but it remains to be seen how doctors will respond to this initiative. A recent survey shows that there is considerable resistance among some GPs to becoming involved with the management of drug users to any extent.

Crisis intervention

The ACMD has also recommended that units should be developed to provide accommodation and care for injecting drug users at times of crisis. Although this is supported by all those involved in drug and AIDS work in Lothian, there is a strong feeling that such centres are needed for *all* serious drug users and not just those who are injecting and are therefore at higher risk of HIV infection. Those agencies, primarily in the voluntary sector, who have been striving for many years to obtain funding for drug projects have reason to be incensed by what they see as a sudden interest in the problem now that AIDS has become an issue. Funding which was previously unavailable has materialised; health services, social services and the Scottish Office are all perceived as taking the problems of drug users on board purely because of AIDS. It is difficult to gainsay this view, and it is regrettable that political differences sometimes obscure the fact that the vast majority of the agencies involved are in agreement about the need for services for drug users.

Specialist initiatives
The City Hospital
One of the more controversial developments in the management of drug use has taken place in the Infectious Diseases Unit of the City Hospital. In the absence of a specialist consultant psychiatrist in drug abuse, the consultants there commenced substitute prescribing in early 1987 in the hope that, by allowing patients who were HIV positive to abstain from injection, this would delay the progression of the disease. As word spread, referrals of other drug users were made to the unit. Although there were medical reasons for some HIV-negative drug users to be accepted for treatment, it became clear that the service would soon be overwhelmed by the demand for help with drug treatment problems. As a result, there is now a policy that only HIV-positive individuals will be prescribed substitute drugs, and there are strict guidelines concerning the prescriptions.

The consultants and staff involved admit to the contradictory nature of the policy, whereby those who are HIV-positive can receive prescribed medication but those who are negative (and therefore still at risk of infection) cannot. However, they have been unable to take any other action, given the volume of work devoted to those who are already infected. Considerable concern has also been expressed about the provision of substitute prescriptions, particularly of Methadone, without specialist psychiatric input. Critics of the service point to the fact that psychiatrists in other parts of the country are responsible for the treatment of drug users, as if this were sufficient reason for refraining from any other kind of intervention in the absence of a specialist psychiatric service in drug use in Edinburgh.

On occasion, in-patient detoxification is carried out within the Infectious Diseases Unit. Usually the individuals are well known to the service and their commitment to the cessation of drug use has been fully assessed.

Treatment is carried out using a behavioural contract and, as far as possible, attempts are made to ensure that adequate social support is provided in the community in order to maximise the possibility of the person remaining drug free after discharge. Nursing staff – already trained and experienced in infectious diseases nursing – are now proficient in helping drug users. Their intervention is crucial in managing drug users on the ward, whether they are admitted for detoxification or for reasons of illness. It is worth noting that this service has evolved satisfactorily without the benefit of formal psychiatric or psychological input.

However proficient the service at the City Hospital, it cannot possibly and should not have had to meet all the needs for drug treatment in Lothian. As the number of ill people with HIV-related disease increases in Lothian, the Infectious Diseases Unit will be less able to deal with drug problems, and so there is a pressing need for alternative services. Psychiatric input is urgently required, not only for expert help in managing drug use, but also in managing the psychiatric manifestations of HIV disease and dementia. The well-publicised link between HIV infection and injecting drug use in Edinburgh sometimes obscures the fact that there are many others infected who will require the help of psychiatric services.

The ACMD commented that many of the measures recommended in the McClelland Report had not been acted upon. The 15-bed unit at the City Hospital is planned to be ready in 1990, at the earliest. Out-patient facilities at that hospital are spartan and are an irritation for staff and patients alike. Day beds are required for pentamidine inhalation, blood transfusions, etc. *now*, but await the upgrading of the out-patient facilities, which is also planned. Counsellors, doctors, nurses, a psychologist, social workers and research staff all share the same 'office' space within the out-patient clinic. Available rooms are almost all equipped as medical consulting rooms and are therefore not particularly suitable for counselling or psychological intervention. The availability of suitable out-patient facilities seems far away and there is considerable frustration over the fact that provision of services is lagging so far behind the problems which are already present. These difficulties highlight how slow the NHS is to provide physical facilities because of the clumsy structure and operation of Health Board, Common Services Agency and contractors.

However, there have been some important developments in the services for drug users in Lothian over the past two years. The voluntary agencies concerned with the problem have received additional funding, there is additional support provided by the Social Work Department, and Lothian Health Board has established the Community Drugs Problem Service.

The Community Drugs Problem Service (CDPS)

The CDPS is in its infancy, having been established only in April 1988, and its efficacy still has to be measured, though this may be difficult when there is not necessarily a consensus about its aims. At present, the CDPS has one consultant psychiatrist who takes referrals from a variety of health service, social work and voluntary agencies. This compares with two consultants for alcohol problems, four for the elderly and eight for general psychiatry. There are also two community psychiatric nurses. Where drug maintenance or reducing doses of drugs is considered appropriate, the individual's GP is asked to prescribe in conjunction with a programme which requires weekly attendance by the drug user. Preliminary indications are that GPs are using the service, and many of the voluntary drug agencies are also actively participating in the programmes. Without their co-operation, the service would be unable to function. It may be that this initiative will help GPs who were previously loath to prescribe to take on the management of drug users themselves. It is clear that many users who were previously injecting have stabilised on substitute prescriptions and have been enabled to give up chaotic lifestyles as well as injecting drug use.

The CDPS received 94 referrals in the first six months of its existence, and 60 drug users attend regularly; of these, most are HIV-negative. The service has already reached the point where a waiting list may have to be instituted. In its first three months, it was able to respond rapidly to referrals, and the good attendance rate presumably reflected this. With a waiting list, there will be many whose desire for help will wane before they can be seen, and there is concern that the optimum opportunity to draw them into treatment may be lost.

It is generally agreed that a system incorporating a walk-in public health clinic, an expanded CDPS and a drug dependency unit with in-patient facilities would be required to manage the drug problem in Lothian effectively. However, it is often unclear where the responsibility for planning these services lies; the Mental Health Unit, the Lothian Health Board and the Scottish Office are generally blamed in ascending order of importance, influence and access to resources. It is perceived, rightly or wrongly, that there is little political motivation to improve services for drug users, although that is a keystone to preventing the further spread of HIV infection in Lothian. It is from that group of people that infection is most likely to spread to the heterosexual non-drug-using community.

Behaviour change

A recent study has indicated that changes have taken place in drug-using behaviour in Edinburgh. Robertson, Skidmore and Roberts (1988b) have followed up a cohort of 49 injecting drug users. They were initially interviewed in 1986, at which time they reported having become aware of the AIDS problem between the end of 1985 and the beginning of 1986. This coincided with media campaigns and the realisation within the professional community that there was a serious problem in Lothian. A follow up of nearly 80 per cent of the subjects after one year showed that there had been a significant decline both in injecting drug use and needle sharing, and in the number of sexual partners among both HIV-positive and HIV-negative users. These data are encouraging, but it is unclear to what extent they generalise outside the particular cohort. For instance, within the area from which they were recruited, there has been particularly successful input from the local drug group. In addition the GPs involved in the study have been more involved in the care and management of drug users than any others in Lothian. As a result, changes in behaviour within this group may not be seen in other areas. The study nevertheless shows that behavioural change is possible within a group often regarded as incapable of change.

Drug use in Lothian has altered considerably since the spread of infection became known. Drug users report that there has been far less heroin available in Edinburgh, and drugs such as Temgesic, temazepam and dihydrocodeine are now more widely used. Unfortunately, the first two are frequently injected, as are other substances, such as other benzodiazepines. Although the availability of injecting equipment has increased, the measures taken to date may not preclude the continued spread of infection through contaminated needles. Efforts to address this problem must be made in tandem with the need to prevent heterosexual transmission.

A study of heterosexual transmission is currently being carried out by the City Hospital, the Muirhouse Medical Group and the Department of Genito-urinary Medicine at the Middlesex Hospital in London. This study is at an early stage, and results are not yet available. However, France *et al.* (1988) reported the results of a study involving 63 people whose only risk factor for infection had been heterosexual intercourse with an individual who was seropositive but clinically well. This differed from other research in that many of these studies concern individuals who had already become ill in some way. In the France study, it was found that one man and six women became infected. All seven had had regular heterosexual intercourse with the infected partner, and all denied having anal intercourse; they had all been in a relationship for 18 months or more. When analysis was confined to confirmed infected drug users in relationships of over 18 months (that is, excluding casual partners), the prevalence of heterosexual transmission was 21 per cent. Perhaps even more alarming was the finding that 12 out of 25 couples interviewed reported that they never used contraceptives; 9 used condoms after discovering that one of the partners was seropositive but only 5 of these always used them.

The combination of a high rate of seroprevalence within the population, the fact that the majority of those who are seropositive are young and heterosexually active, that there is evidence that condom use is limited and that the data in the above study may refer to a group who are relatively less infectious than those who are clinically unwell leads many people working in the area to believe that the next phase of the Lothian epidemic will be through heterosexual transmission. This may not only be a problem for

Edinburgh, as the ACMD pointed out: many drug users move around Britain and the spread of HIV in Scotland will lead to the virus spreading more rapidly throughout the UK.

The human side

All the foregoing, academic in nature, should not be allowed to obscure the human suffering which this epidemic is engendering among whole families and communities in Edinburgh. Dr Roy Robertson (personal communication) has pointed out that some families have two, three or four infected members. The first fatalities in the cohort of the Edinburgh Drug Addiction Study were the suicide of an HIV-positive ex-drug user and the death from AIDS of a mother who had tried heroin a few times with her son, an infected user. The first diagnosed case of pneumocystis was in a heterosexual contact of a drug user. Of those seen at the various clinics, probably 50 per cent who are no longer using 'hard drugs' stopped doing so before they discovered that they were infected. Many have settled down, married and had children. They may live with the fear that their partners and children may become infected; their partners fear for their husbands and wives as well as for themselves and their children. The drug-using population is often difficult to help for various reasons, but that should not obscure the fact that some are responsible, are capable of making changes and are as caring of their loved ones as any other member of the population.

Case study 1
Mrs A. has three children, aged 12, 8 and 2. She became HIV-positive through intermittent injecting drug use in 1984. She has not taken any drugs for four years, and found that she was antibody-positive only a year ago. Her husband, who was so violent towards her that she tried to escape him on numerous occasions, continued to use drugs and is currently in prison. She has moved away from her community, family and friends in the hope that he will be unable to find her and the children when he is released. He does not know whether or not he is antibody-positive, but maintains that, if he is, it will be because she infected him. Her 2-year-old daughter is being monitored and, although the child no longer has HIV antibodies, Mrs A. is still afraid that she will become ill. She has told only one person that she is infected with HIV and is terrified of others finding out as she is afraid that her children will be ostracised. She lives a lonely, isolated existence, frightened of what will happen when her husband is released, and of what will happen to her children if she becomes ill and dies. Her main expressed concern is that the children should not be separated or given into the custody of their father if anything happens to her.

The children

The presence of a large number of infected heterosexual young people has also meant that there has been a relatively high number of births to infected mothers. There are now 53 children in Lothian born to infected mothers, although it remains unclear how many of these are themselves infected with the virus. Many were antibody-positive at birth but by 18 months showed no antibody evidence, maternal antibody having cleared (Peckham *et al.*, 1988). It is believed that the rate of infectivity and maternal foetal transmission may increase as some mothers become unwell and therefore possibly more infectious.

The service for children was set up in January 1986 when it was realised that three babies had been born to antibody-positive mothers. At that time, it was believed that 50–60 per cent of these children would die. The MRC, an AIDS charity and Lothian Health Board have funded, respectively, a research fellow, a technician and a health visitor to help with the care of the children. To date it appears that 20–30 per cent of the children are infected, but this prevalence rate may well rise.

There is good co-operation between this team and both the maternity services and the social work department, who may provide foster care if necessary. Such fostering is more often required because the parents and children are multiply deprived than because of HIV itself. Some children have become ill and are treated with zidovudine or immunoglobulin. It is too early to make predictions about the direct effect of HIV, or of treatment, on these children, and it is hoped that the European Collaborative Study, which includes the data from Lothian, will provide further knowledge over the next few years.

General practitioners' response

As in other areas of clinical practice, GPs in Lothian have tended to work in isolation in their own practices, dealing with the problems of the HIV epidemic which confront them as effectively as they can. The opportunity, time, energy and expertise to audit their own activity, let alone consider how others are coping, are not very often available. While GPs sometimes react against advice from others, this problem has not occurred because local advice on tackling HIV infection and its prevention has been largely absent. Of course, for many, actual infection is indeed someone else's problem, but GPs are short sighted if they neither care how their colleagues are coping nor expect to have some preventive role themselves.

The difficulties faced by GPs in Lothian were discussed by the Local Medical Committee (LMC), but there has been no obvious move to influence the situation. The chairman did write to all GPs suggesting that they do not prescribe large quantities of addictive drugs and that they avoid prescribing Temgesic which is known to be injected by drug users.

The issue of leadership of general practitioners by general practitioners is not peculiar to the problems of HIV infection. The LMC does not see itself as offering leadership on any matter. As the GP Subcommittee of the Area Medical Committee (in Scotland, the Health Boards fulfil the role of the FPCs in England), it advises the Lothian Health Board. The Area Medical Committee, too, has had little to say on preventive strategy for this new problem. Similarly, there has been little obvious activity from the local faculty of the Royal College of General Practitioners.

A group of GPs did meet together in January 1988 to exchange information and ideas, derive support and learn from each other. The Lothian Health Board AIDS co-ordinator, the CDPS psychiatrist and the AIDS service psychologist now meet with them monthly, in the evening. This group initially shared their varying perceptions of the size and nature of the problem confronting all members in their own surgeries. Difficulties within partnerships were aired and clinical management debated. Unsurprisingly, approaches to the management of drug users came up frequently. It was agreed that some educational initiative for GPs should be attempted and the blessing of the LMC for this was sought and received. It commenced in October 1988 and initially took the form of a questionnaire to assess unmet needs and provoke thought. This was followed by a series of six fortnightly information sheets dealing with aspects of the Lothian HIV problem, under the title of 'Local AIDS'.

There are a number of important issues for GPs in Lothian in addressing the problems of HIV infection. Those discussed below are primarily concerned with the difficulties of dealing with drug users within the general practice setting.

The preventive role

Some GPs wish to offer a primary care service to drug users but remain sceptical of their power to influence drug-using behaviour significantly. Yet if GPs are to help limit the spread of HIV, regular contact with the infected group and those most at risk, including injecting drug users, will be an important contribution.

When a new clinical entity appears on the scene, GPs often expect to learn and do learn from their specialist colleagues in hospital on a case-to-case basis. This serves individual patients well enough if they are seen at the hospital, have an identifiable problem to be learned about and are known to the GP. The mode by which GPs adopt and adapt aspects of preventive health-care and health promotion in a novel situation seems less clear. Lack of a coherent preventive policy, promoted both from hospital and at Health Board level, has been a marked weakness in Lothian.

Although the childhood immunisation programme and cervical screening are both computerised by the Health Board, there remains doubt in the minds of some GPs about the usefulness of such preventive programmes. The public so often seem unaffected by advice offered during consultations. Prevention and health education are tackled in general practice but most comfortably when GPs are confident of the message they wish to convey and are at ease with their patients. The fact that many local GPs neither feel comfortable with injecting drug users nor believe that they have the knowledge to treat them is an important issue.

Lack of familiarity with the problems

Drug users are still seen as a time-consuming complication in the day-to-day business of providing primary care to a population of whom they are a minority. No doctor wants to be 'conned' into prescribing drugs of addiction which may be added to the pool of prescribed drugs in the city available to be misused. This fear may pervade a consultation, fuelled in the past by intermittent presentations of 'temporary residents' with stories of chronic pain that is only relieved by opiate analgesics and benzodiazepines. Most GPs know that hospital out-patient and in-patient facilities, already limited, have been reluctantly offered to drug users only to be rejected by them because the service offered was inappropriate to their needs. Local practitioners, willing to take on such patients, have faced the thankless task of trying to meet the medical needs of this group without the optimism, skills, experience and backup needed to address the main problem of drug dependence. Perhaps not surprisingly, the norm has been a rigid service with no prescribing, some surgeries actively discouraging injecting drug users from registering or removing them from their lists after the minimum three months. There has been, after all, little incentive to provide a service given that (*a*) many of these individuals are difficult, undisciplined and hostile (and some are aggressive and violent) and (*b*) there have been such poor backup services.

Prescribing practice

It is true to say that the medical care of drug users would be much more acceptable to GPs if it were not for the thorny issue of prescriptions. Almost inevitably a consultation becomes a discussion, if not an argument, about what should or should not be prescribed, and real health issues may be obscured.

In general, there are three different approaches which GPs may adopt with regard to the management of the drug user, and particularly with regard to maintenance prescribing. First, they can make a policy decision that drugs, whether opiates or benzodiazepines, are never prescribed to those whom they suspect of drug use on a serious scale. Second, they can opt for prescribing what the patients ask for because this precludes exhausting arguments about the need for drugs in general, the kind of drug in particular and the required dosage. The third, and hardest, option is undoubtedly that of attempting to prescribe sensibly, bearing in mind individual needs, in an attempt to stabilise the patient, to preclude the use of illegally bought and possibly contaminated drugs and, most importantly now, to reduce the risk of injection and infection. No one would deny that this is difficult to get right, that overdoses occur even with legally obtained drugs and that there is leakage of legally prescribed drugs on to the illicit market. These are serious concerns for GPs and, as a result, it is unsurprising that many opt for having as little as possible to do with drug users.

The significant exception to the above has been the involvement of the Muirhouse Medical Group, based in the north of Edinburgh amid several large council housing estates. Within this group, a flexible, responsive and usually overburdened general practice service has been offered for drug users. In addition, the information obtained through the practice and published in the Edinburgh Drug Addiction Study has generated valuable information about levels of infection and the behaviour of drug users.

Two of the partnership of six doctors have become most identified with the treatment of the drug users. They have demonstrated an all-round concern for these individuals, combined with a willingness to prescribe maintenance and reduction medication long before this had become an even marginally acceptable practice within medical circles in Lothian. The other partners in the practice have preferred not to prescribe in the same way and only encounter drug users when covering the practice out of hours and during holidays. This divergence of opinion and prescribing practice within partnerships of GPs is echoed elsewhere. Whether partnerships can successfully cope with such differences in such contentious areas of clinical practice is becoming an increasingly important issue.

Patient load
In Lothian's largely urban setting, there is a concentration of drug users and, therefore, of antibody-positive patients in certain locations. Table 9 shows

Table 9 **Estimates of the numbers of HIV-positive patients registered in 56 practices in Lothian Region**

Estimate	*Number of practices*
Fewer than 2 patients per 1,000	39
Between 1 and 3 per 1,000	12
More than 3 per 1,000	4
More than 10 per 1,000	1

the results of an informal survey, carried out in 1988, of 56 practices in Lothian with registers comprising a total of 400,000 patients. GPs were asked to estimate the number of HIV-positive individuals registered in their practices.

There are questions about the sharing of the load between practices and whether the more heavily burdened practices can cope with their preventive primary care and, ultimately, terminal care responsibilities for this group. How effective GPs can be without additional resources and training is also unknown.

For those doctors who have seen fit to incorporate the prescribing of opiates in their management of injecting drug users, an increase in workload seems almost inevitable. This increase is related to the need to supervise prescribed drug taking and is largely unconnected with the HIV antibody status of patients. The arguments concerning the desirability of prescribing for both HIV-negative and HIV-positive drug users are well aired elsewhere and need not be expanded here at any length. In prescribing oral drugs for those who are HIV-negative, it is hoped to limit injecting use and therefore the possibility of infection through needle sharing. For those who are HIV-positive, it is hoped the cessation of injecting use will slow down progression of the disease. These hypotheses are almost impossible to prove but appear sufficiently plausible that many doctors are willing to embark upon prescribing which they might have otherwise found unacceptable.

Of course, the attempt to stop drug injection or at least reduce sharing of needles and syringes need not include prescribing. For some time, some GPs have been providing sterile syringes and needles as well as condoms to those who are at a risk, in line with McClelland Report recommendations. Regular consultation, which includes discussion of equipment and/or prescription provision, may in itself help the drug users to develop a more beneficial relationship with the GP and therefore make it more likely that the guilt/demand axis is removed from the relationship.

There is no doubt, however, that the burden of extra consultations, inappropriate demands and phone calls in between fixed consultations remains a problem and a disincentive to those who might consider sharing the load by accepting individuals belonging to this group of patients. At the moment, the load is unacceptably heavy for practices within specific locations in Edinburgh. It appears that, in most cases, more than ten injecting drug users per partner imposes a load which can threaten the balance of work and may detract from the service available to other patients. Table 10 gives current figures for two different practices in Edinburgh and thus some indication of the problems faced.

The smaller practice experiences similar problems to that of Muirhouse, albeit on a smaller scale. Patients rub shoulders in the restricted space of the waiting-room, and it is only too evident that their lifestyles are totally

Table 10 Injecting drug users attending practices in (a) a 'high-risk' area of council estates and (b) a central Edinburgh 'mixed community'

	(a) Muirhouse	(b) North Central
Patient List	10,800	2,468
Partners	7	2
Total weekly appointments	700	155
HIV-positive registered	55	6
IDUs seen regularly	105	10
IDUs' appointments weekly	55	8

different and incompatible. The two partners have growing experience of HIV infection and drug use, but one partner sees nearly all the injecting drug users. Consultations with them occupy 10 per cent of his weekly appointments, and this affects his general availability to others. It is freely acknowledged that mistakes have been made, and policies remain under discussion. Receptionists have been stressed and made anxious by over-demanding and unreasonable individuals. The second partner genuinely doubts that much can be achieved by the more flexible approach which has been adopted. On the contrary, he feels that there may be losses to the practice as a whole, a concern which is undoubtedly shared, with reason, by other practices which take on drug users.

In order to devote time and energy to the problem, GPs may have to cease doing something else in the practice. They need to be convinced that the problem is real and important enough for such a redistribution of efforts to be considered worthwhile. They would be foolish to forget their duty to their whole patient population as well as to themselves, their partners and their families to remain well and maintain a satisfactory general practice business.

Communication

The general problem of communication between hospital services and GPs is explored elsewhere, but specific problems about communication have arisen in the context of the drug-using population.

The commencement of oral Methadone prescribing at the City Hospital in early 1987 was not widely known, although GPs were notified about individual patients. The City Hospital's decision to begin this was born out of frustration that nothing appeared to be being done about the continuing possibility of infection through injecting drug use. The likely controversy over the new policy undoubtedly led to its introduction without publicity, but many GPs felt aggrieved that there had been little or no discussion about it and that they were sometimes left 'holding the baby'. It is of utmost importance in such a situation that decisions about prescribing be communicated rapidly between the different medical agencies. In Lothian, there were complaints from both sides that this communication did not occur, and that this, in some cases, led to multiple prescribing.

Further problems in communication arose because of the lack of computerised records which resulted in delays in new patients' records catching up with them. For patients with HIV infection or a history of drug use and treatment, early access to past information is especially helpful. A more rapid telephone service from Lothian Health Board exists, but this stretches staff-time even more, and it is discouraging to be asked to limit such requests because of staff shortages.

The development of the Community Drugs Problem Service may help to ease some of the difficulties which have been evident in the past. GPs are now more directly involved in the treatment of drug users, are in control of the issue of prescriptions and have a point of reference from which they can receive both support and advice. The factors mentioned earlier which are already putting the CPDS under pressure could cause further problems if GPs discover that they have taken on the care of drug users only to find that the present minimal service is unable to provide adequate backup.

Overall, there is little doubt that GPs will be heavily involved in the care of drug users and HIV-infected people in the future, particularly as the currently infected population becomes ill. It is essential that the initiatives of the GP Group are encouraged, and that GPs are given, not just advice, but also practical help in counselling and caring for their patients. Whether they like it or not, the problems of HIV infection will impinge on practitioners' lives even if they are unwilling to take on the management of drug users.

Case study 2

Mr B. had been a practice patient for several years, and most of his injecting drug use occurred long ago. In 1986, he attended his GP to ask for hepatitis and HIV tests because his dentist wished to have those results before he extracted a tooth. The GP, unfamiliar with HIV problems, agreed and, assuming that the results would be negative, allowed the patient to phone in for his results. These, as it turned out, were positive. When Mr B. phoned the practice, he was told to come in for an appointment. He then stayed away but, a fortnight later, attended about other concerns. His initial anger was replaced by a more optimistic outlook, and the GP was able to persuade him to attend the City Hospital.

His live-in girlfriend was found to be antibody-negative. This has led them to consider the possibility of having a child as, although the girlfriend may get infected on becoming pregnant, there would only be a 25 per cent chance of their baby being infected. He is seen by his GP every two to three weeks, but he continues to turn up late for his appointments. He is prescribed moderate doses of dihydrocodeine and temazepam and is able to work casually in his trade. One of his brothers has AIDS and another is HIV-positive and asymptomatic. He knows about spread by needle sharing and has avoided doing so on the few occasions that he has injected. He is provided with condoms from his GP, and he and his girlfriend are receiving counselling from the hospital services.

The Prison Service

Saughton, the prison in Edinburgh, houses approximately 600 male prisoners with about 5,000 new admissions per year. As well as being the local prison for Edinburgh, and containing a large number of remand prisoners, there are also quite a few long-term prisoners from all parts of the country. Prior to the emergence of HIV infection, a significant number of prisoners had been identified as infected with or carrying the hepatitis B virus, which may be associated with drug use. By the latter part of 1985, the number of new admissions to the prison who confessed to regular use of drugs was declining. The accuracy of this is verified, to an extent, by the strip search that all new prisoners undergo, at which venepuncture marks can be spotted by nursing officers. Changes in sentencing policy, a move towards oral prescribed drugs and away from injectables and maturing out of drug use may all have contributed to this. The part-time medical officer to the prison considers the last explanation the most likely and reckons that the trend will continue, with relatively few cases of drug withdrawal now being observed.

Drug use

Incidents when prisoners are found under the influence of drugs are uncommon. Drugs can easily be brought into the prison, either through open visits or when prisoners are involved in activities outside the prison as part of their rehabilitation process. At present, even prisoners who have been regularly prescribed hypnotics by their GPs in the community are not given these once in prison. There are probably a small number of needles and syringes in the prisoners' hands, although prisoners' tales of their multiple use seem not to be confirmed by prison officers. There are usually between 70 and 80 prisoners who are known to have used drugs or still to be using drugs.

HIV infection

At any one time, about 20 men in the prison are known to be HIV-positive, but it is estimated that another 36 might be infected unknown to the prison staff and, in some cases, unknown to the prisoners themselves. To date, 190 tests have been performed, the vast majority reporting as antibody-positive. Some prisoners have had symptoms and show signs of disease progression, but none so far has had AIDS. While confidentiality is a potential problem, antibody testing is now encouraged.

Saughton prison differs from those in England and Wales in that there is no segregation of infected prisoners, and staff are expected to take appropriate precautions in all circumstances. Those known to be infected receive the required help for medical problems. Improving communication between prisoners and staff, including prison doctors, while preserving an appropriate level of confidentiality is an important issue. Widening that confidentiality to include information to and from the prisoners' GPs could be helpful, as would general information about the availavility of services in the community when such prisoners are released.

Education

A continuing problem is how best to increase awareness of HIV and AIDS without causing undue panic in either staff or inmates. The initial response from the prison department was to issue clear guidelines on hygiene, and, somewhat later, a video was produced and shown to inmates and staff on a few occasions. At an early stage, staff expressed a great deal of concern about handling HIV-positive prisoners. This has largely settled, and anxiety is now only aroused by specific incidents. Proposals for more health education in 1987 were only accepted to the extent that those known to be infected are now offered regular counselling and medical checks, which have been generally well received. There is a continuing need for staff education and support similar to that needed in nursing, medical, educational, social work and other agencies.

New skills and additional resources, combined with better liaison with outside agencies, are all required. The provision of these has begun slowly. In conjunction with the Lothian Health Board, a counselling course for staff is now also being offered. The idea of counselling is a new one among the prison nursing staff, but they are taking on the new role and are now receiving regular updates about HIV and AIDS. All prisoners do not receive regular health education; the notion that showing a video constitutes adequate health promotion is clearly erroneous. Misconceptions among prisoners about infectivity still cause the occasional case of ostracism of those discovered to be antibody-positive. More resources, staff and time are required to do the job of health promotion properly, and the delay in producing these is regrettable. An interdisciplinary AIDS group which meets fortnightly was established in November 1988 within the prison to address these matters.

Preventing the spread of infection

Two practical methods to reduce the spread of infection are practised in the community but still resisted by prison authorities. Provision of sterile needles and syringes is generally thought inappropriate in that environment, but the case for the provision of condoms appears strong and seems to be gaining ground; the ACMD report certainly recommended that it should be given urgent consideration. Still prison governors insist that prison is a 'public place' under the law and so homosexual acts are therefore illegal and cannot be condoned or assisted. This impasse and the rigid guidelines on what is and is not prescribed for prisoners remain under debate.

Scotland's prisons have had exceptionally difficult times recently, and allegations of protection rackets inside, extending to enmesh ex-prisoners and families outside, have been made. The supply of drugs and their continued illicit use in prison, especially when injected, is of great concern. There is little incentive for drug users themselves to deny tales of the insensitivity of prison officers or stories that three contaminated needles are circulating in the Edinburgh's prison. However, it is probably true to say that the issues of testing and counselling are now sensitively and intelligently handled but that preventive measures lag behind. Saughton prison, in its recent liaison with outside agencies, both statutory and voluntary, has certainly taken major strides forward in tackling the problem.

Summary

Projections suggest that 78 people will die from AIDS in Lothian in 1991 (Tayler Report, 1987). Lothian Health Board's report (1988) for the AIDS Control Act emphasises that this will be the major cause of death in the age group 15–44 years – more than deaths from cancer or road traffic accidents. The success of prevention practised now will almost certainly determine whether the annual figure for deaths from AIDS rises or falls during the next decade.

While the problems of treating those with symptoms are complex enough, without any cure in sight, planning and executing a programme of prevention and health promotion in this medical, ethical and social minefield is even more difficult. It is acknowledged that health education in Lothian has been inadequate. The problems in implementing effective health promotion are not new, but the implications of delay and prevarication in tackling the spread of the human immunodeficiency virus are alarming.

In Lothian, the first response has been to offer hospital facilities to those who are infected and those who think that they might be infected. This was a natural consequence of the discovery in 1985 that there was already a large pool of infected individuals. It is understandable that health promotion measures have lagged behind, given the extent of the existing problem. The need to cater for the medical and psychological needs of those infected must be balanced against the need to ensure that HIV infection does not spread further.

The initiatives already taken to reduce or eliminate needle sharing must be actively pursued and extended if this mode of transmission is to be curtailed. Although needle exchanges, pharmacy sales and GP provision of clean equipment are already helping, it is clear that only a limited number of individuals are being reached. The vast majority are probably not in contact with services, and there are distressing accounts from those who are in contact that young people are continuing to embark on injecting drug use including needle sharing.

The weak service for drug users, which has been in existence for a number of years, requires that expertise and experience are borrowed from other areas where there are better established services. Although the Lothian Region and non-statutory agencies are also involved in this, it is generally perceived that responsibility for filling this gap rests with the Health Board and its medical advisers. However, there is a danger that the most obvious and publicised aspects of the epidemic in Lothian – that of the high level of infection among drug users – may lead to a dangerous complacency among the general population, who are probably at greater risk from HIV infection, through heterosexual activity, than in any other area in the UK. There has undoubtedly been a recent increase in the number of relatively new cases of heterosexual infection, and there is urgent need for health education in this area.

Public education on a large scale is still required in Lothian. Messages about AIDS were hard to avoid in public places in London in 1987; in Lothian, they have always been hard to find. If heterosexual spread is to be controlled in this area, where an estimated 1 per cent of the young male population is already infected, AIDS must be presented to the public as something which does concern them and is relevant to their sexual behaviour.

Statutory and non-statutory organisations have changed gear to address the problem, and all are doing their best to promote health and prevent the spread of infection, but, to date, there has been too little co-ordination of such efforts. Committees have formed to gather and share information and to plan services, but strategy remains unclear. Delay in taking action on recommendations has been disappointing, but plans have eventually come to fruition. There is always the concern that the plans are made one step behind the problem rather than in anticipation of the future course of the epidemic. The evidence which is necessary to shape policy continues to change, but that is no good reason for delay.

It is accepted that there are inconsistencies in the messages which the caring professions must promote. We want people to stop injecting but will provide syringes and needles for them. In the area of sexual transmission, we strongly advise against anal intercourse but provide condoms for homosexual men. We advise against pregnancy for those who are HIV-positive but help them to achieve childbirth if they wish. The issues surrounding harm reduction are difficult, but in Lothian they have generally been faced by individual professionals much earlier and tackled more effectively than by those in higher management. Initiatives, such as those at the City Hospital, in Muirhouse and in the establishment of the Community Drugs Problem Service, have been driven by specific individuals, rather than by governmental, regional, Health Board or social service policy.

On an individual level, GPs, family planning centres and agencies who are in a position to advise about sexual behaviour must extend their efforts to discuss AIDS as an issue which potentially touches everyone. The brunt of the work with those at risk in general practice has been borne by a minority of GPs. Gradually, as patients have moved and as GPs have gained confidence, the load is being shared. Experience in handling those already infected produces a facility and an urgency to promote safe behaviour and healthy lifestyles with others less at risk. Officials at the Scottish Home and Health Department are discussing with the British Medical Association in Scotland how resources may be targeted in general practice. This will not be easy. However, for those in general practice whose work has expanded to encompass preventive measures, who have high numbers of patients at risk and who have been willing to take on the care of drug users, specialist and more general assistance will be helpful.

In all areas of care and health promotion, we need to look closely at our performance to date. The load on agencies is not equally divided and there is a need for much more sharing of information. Insights from hospitals to community, community to prisons and so on are important. The introduction of new workers into this field should be a strengthening rather than diluting change. Additional expertise and replacements will be required; for many individuals, the work has taken time far beyond a normal commitment to their work. Key people must not be allowed to 'burn out' quietly while everyone else works away in his/her own corner. The pace of spread and the progression of the disease has led to a feeling of urgency among the involved professions which is productive, but they frequently find themselves following rather than leading as the epidemic changes.

As Lothian enters its fourth year of awareness of the high prevalence of infection locally, strategy needs to be further identified. As AIDS inevitably becomes a bigger problem, the prevention of spread must retain its priority in the face of the needs of those already infected. The balance of provision for treatment and prevention may be difficult because of the level of infection in Lothian. Health promotion groups, the Royal College of General Practitioners and the Faculty of Community Medicine share a responsibility with local authorities and health boards to ensure that they maintain momentum and that their educational initiatives are fresh and targeted appropriately. What we learn and what we do about this epidemic should stand us in good stead to tackle other aspects of care in a more co-ordinated and effective manner.

Acknowledgements
We would like to thank Dr David Jolliffe (medical officer at Saughton Prison), Dr Roy Robertson, Dr Jackie Mok and all other colleagues in Lothian who gave advice and assistance.

Tables 6 and 7 are derived from data made available by the Communicable Disease (Scotland) Unit.

References

Brettle, R. P., Bisset, K., Burns, S. *et al.* (1987) Human immunodeficiency virus and drug misuse: the Edinburgh experience. *British Medical Journal*, 295, 421–4.

Department of Health & Social Security. (1988) *AIDS and Drug Misuse.* Report by the Advisory Council on the Misuse of Drugs (Part 1). London, HMSO.

France, A. J., Skidmore, C. A., Robertson, J. R. *et al.* (1988) Heterosexual spread of human immunodeficiency virus in Edinburgh. *British Medical Journal*, 296, 526–9.

Lothian Health Board. (1988) *AIDS in Lothian: Everyone's Concern.* Report in response to the Health Service Management AIDS (Control) Act 1987.

McClelland, D. B. L. (chairman). (1986) *HIV Infection in Scotland.* Report of the Scottish Committee on HIV Infection and Intravenous Drug Misuse. Edinburgh, Scottish Home and Health Department.

Peckham, C. S., Senturia, Y. D., Ades, A. E. *et al.* (1988) Mother-to-child transmission of HIV infection (report from the European Collaborative Study). *The Lancet*, iii, 1039–43.

Peutherer, J. F., Edmond, E., Simmonds, P. *et al.* (1985) HTLV111 antibody in Edinburgh drug addicts. *The Lancet*, ii, 1129–30.

Robertson, J. R., Bucknall, A. B. V., Welsby, P. D. *et al.* (1986) An epidemic of AIDS-related virus infection amongst intravenous drug abusers in a Scottish general practice. *British Medical Journal*, 292, 527–9.

Robertson, J. R., Skidmore, C. A. and Roberts, J. J. K. (1988a) The dynamics of an illicit drug scene. *Scottish Medical Journal*, 33, No. 4, 293.

Robertson, J. R., Skidmore, C. A. and Roberts, J. J. K. (1988b) HIV infection in intravenous drug users: a follow-up study indicating changes in risk-taking behaviour. *British Journal of Addiction*, 83, 387–91.

Tayler, W. J. (chairman). (1987) *Report of the National Scottish Working Party on Health Service Implications of HIV Infection.* Edinburgh, HMSO.

Scottish Health Authorities' Priorities for the Eighties (The SHAPE Report). (1985) Scottish Home and Health Department, Edinburgh, HMSO.

Working Together: The response to AIDS in Brighton

Dr Angela Iverson, Simon Cavicchia and Dr Gordon R. Macphail

Brighton Health District is geographically the smallest of three district health authorities in East Sussex, but the 301,000 people resident in it (1981 census) comprised just over half of the population of the whole area. Of that number, 23 per cent were over 65 years of age. The population is concentrated in the coastal areas of Brighton, Hove and Newhaven, with Lewes, the county town and administrative centre, some nine miles inland.

Brighton Health Authority is surrounded by Mid-Downs Health Authority to the north, Eastbourne Health Authority to the east and Worthing Health Authority to the west. Brighton is a thriving holiday resort, and the population of the town increases substantially during the summer months. It has also established itself as a commercial and administrative centre with a large number of office developments and relocations in recent years. There is no significant immigrant population, and the social class breakdown is weighted towards social classes 1 and 2, with an overall morbidity and mortality experience favourable in comparison with national averages. Brighton has a large gay community, with an active local gay scene.

Organisational structures

Brighton Health District is one of 15 districts in the South East Thames Region. The areas governed by Brighton and Hove borough councils are entirely within the district boundary, as is that of Lewes District Council with the exception of Seaford and East Blatchington which are in Eastbourne Health District. Brighton Borough Council is Labour controlled, Hove and Lewes are Conservative controlled and the East Sussex County Council has a minority Conservative administration. However, all four Members of Parliament are Conservative.

The voluntary sector within the district is strong in the field of HIV infection and AIDS; this is discussed in a later section. Housing associations are also playing a leading role in provision for people with AIDS.

The East Sussex Family Practitioner Committee is responsible for the provision of primary care services. Only 14 per cent of GPs are single handed, and 1.5 per cent of GPs are over 70 years of age. There are seven training practices within Brighton Health District.

There is a large active Health Promotion Department within the health district, and Manpower Services Commission workers are also employed.

Joint planning arrangements are outlined below in Figure 9. The AIDS Liaison Group, which meets quarterly, provides a forum for all agencies involved in the prevention of the spread of HIV infection and in the care and treatment of those infected with the virus. Information can be exchanged, and targets set for further inter-agency co-operation. The group ensures that the needs of people with HIV infection can be communicated to local and district joint planning teams. An important task for this group is co-ordination of the health promotion programme for HIV infection, and a sub-group of the officers and representatives involved has been set up. The membership of the AIDS Liaison Group consists of:

Brighton Health Authority
County council social services and education departments
Borough/district council environmental health officers
Voluntary organisations
Terrence Higgins Trust
Sussex AIDS Centre and Helpline
Brighton & Hove Community Health Council

Figure 9 **Joint planning forums in Brighton Health District**

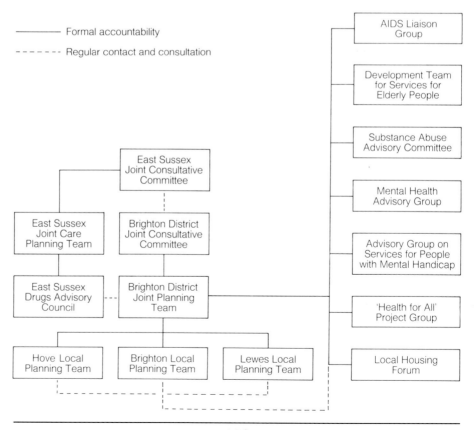

East Sussex Family Practitioner Committee
Tarner & Coppercliff Nursing Homes
Local churches

South East Thames has a Regional AIDS Action Group which meets at regular intervals; it comprises representatives from statutory and voluntary agencies. The Regional Health Authority has organised study days on AIDS/HIV infection, and there is a regional training adviser.

There is a tradition of commitment to intersectoral co-operation with Brighton District, examples of which are a successful mental handicap community care project and a variety of health promotion projects. In the field of AIDS/HIV infection, co-operation between statutory and voluntary agencies has developed well.

General hospital services

The majority of general hospital services are provided on two sites: the Royal Sussex County Hospital, the main acute hospital in the district, and Brighton General Hospital, both of which are located in Brighton. There are plans to relocate, in part, some of the services provided by these hospitals in a new hospital to be built in Hove. However, there are a large number of other hospitals, and in-patient care for people with HIV infection and AIDS has been provided at two of these, with out-patient care at a further four hospitals and drug dependency and general psychiatric treatment at other sites. Co-ordinating care and treatment policies is made difficult by these geographical factors.

Brighton is within easy commuting distance of London. The main London teaching hospitals – especially the Middlesex, St Stephen's and St Mary's – have attracted a proportion of Brighton residents with HIV infection. Travelling presents more problems for these people when they become ill.

The prevalence of HIV infection and AIDS

As of 31 October 1988, the cumulative number of people diagnosed with AIDS was 55 (Table 11), of whom 33 are known to have died.

Table 11 Numbers of people with AIDS diagnosed in the Brighton Health Authority

	1984	1
	1985	5
	1986	8
	1987	20
Jan–Oct	1988	21

The Sussex AIDS Centre and Helpline are aware of an additional 20 individuals with AIDS who attend London centres for treatment.

HIV antibody-positive results and test requests are collated on a monthly basis by the Genito-urinary Medicine (GUM) Clinic, which sends a return to the Authority's Department of Community Medicine. The figures are then sent to the Borough Environmental Health Officer in Brighton for inclusion in a regular Environmental Health Committee report, and are therefore routinely made available to the public.

The cumulative number of Brighton Health District residents who are known to be HIV antibody-positive by the GUM clinic is 259. In addition, there are 20 individuals who were diagnosed and are treated in Brighton, but who are resident outside the health district. In the year between 1 April 1987 and 31 March 1988, 3,616 HIV antibody tests were carried out by the Public Health Laboratory. One quarter of these requests originated from outside the health district, a quarter were from the GUM clinic and drug dependency unit, and half were from local GPs. The high proportion of test requests from GPs may be due to the great awareness of HIV infection by the large gay community in Brighton. The majority of those tested and found to be positive in Brighton are homosexual/bisexual males.

Injecting drug use
Since March 1986, all new referrals to the drug dependency unit in Brighton have been offered HIV antibody testing:

March 1986–March 1987: 211 new referrals offered testing, of whom 127 accepted and 6 were HIV antibody-positive

March 1987–May 1988: 150 new referrals offered testing of whom 34 accepted and 5 were HIV antibody-positive

The reduction in the proportion accepting testing is related to the introduction of pre-test counselling, and greater awareness of the drawbacks of testing among the client group.

In addition, contact tracing revealed 7 further positive individuals, three of whom are babies. One-third of all the HIV antibody-positive individuals known to the drug dependency unit have come from abroad: Spain, Italy, Holland and France. Injecting drug users comprised 7 per cent of known HIV antibody-positive people as of 31 March 1988, but this proportion may increase in the future.

Response to the problem

Initial impact
As early as 1983, the Brighton Gay Switchboard and Brighton Gay Community Organisation were preparing leaflets and briefing papers about

AIDS, and asking the health authority what plans were available to cope with an increased number of cases.

In May 1983, consideration was first given in the health district to the need to review control-of-infection guidelines because of concern over the newly described 'acquired immune deficiency syndrome'. In October 1983, the first person with AIDS was seen in Brighton, and the Consultant in Genito-urinary Medicine asked the District Medical Officer to set up a committee urgently to consider the problem.

A small grant was made by the health district to the Brighton Gay Switchboard in April 1984. At the same time, guidelines on the management of AIDS patients were first drafted by a small group comprising a consultant physician, consultant in genito-urinary medicine, specialist in community medicine and the director of the Public Health Laboratory. The following month, the Brighton Gay Switchboard offered to participate in staff training within the health district.

By June 1984, guidelines on the management of AIDS patients had been circulated by the District Medical Officer to the Medical Cogwheel Division and the District Hospital Medical Committee and to nurse and unit management.

In September 1984, a person with AIDS, having discharged himself from hospital, needed care in the community. The policy prior to this had stated that community nurses would not be involved in caring for people with AIDS, but this had to be changed and, naturally, the nursing staff were concerned about personal safety. Production of nursing guidelines coincided with the identification of viral aetiology, and community nurses were then prepared to take on the care of people with AIDS. Counselling relating to HIV antibody testing was considered in 1984.

From July 1985 onwards, AIDS services have developed in response to funds made available from the DHSS allocation to regions.

Structural responses

The AIDS Working Party was set up early in 1984. The group was and is convened by the District Medical Officer/Specialist in Community Medicine.

The AIDS Working Party is a free-standing health service group which considers service provision and funding, the development of specific policies and guidelines, and health promotion issues. A small sub-group meets occasionally to discuss issues related to the use of zidovudine.

Planning for hospital and community services is the responsibility of the AIDS Working Party, whereas planning for home care, primary care and health promotion activities takes place mainly within the AIDS Liaison Group (part of the joint planning arrangements).

Although there may seem to be a plethora of groups, in practice they work efficiently. In particular, the AIDS Liaison Group has developed into a useful forum for the exchange of views and information between the voluntary and statutory agencies.

Policy responses

A district AIDS strategy is in preparation, and will be a jointly agreed statement by all agencies and organisations represented on the AIDS Liaison Group. The strategy has been developed by the Department of Community Medicine.

The district AIDS policy had a long gestation as draft documents went out to consultation several times. The policy, which has only recently been endorsed by the health authority, is comprehensive and covers in-patient, out-patient and community care, counselling, testing, employment and confidentiality issues. AIDS has highlighted the difficulties involved in providing clinical waste collection and disposal services for people in the community. Control of AIDS infection guidelines are updated by the consultant microbiologist. The AIDS policy itself is updated by the Specialist in Community Medicine (Environmental Health) (SCM [EH]) who is the AIDS co-ordinator within the district, and chairs the AIDS Working Party and the Liaison Group.

Funding and resources

Separate funds for AIDS have been allocated by the South East Thames Region. In previous years, these funds were limited, and most expenditure on AIDS was met from existing budgets. In 1988/9, the allocation has been more substantial, and reflects the costs of caring for people with HIV infection and with AIDS. The SCM (EH) is responsible for producing the annual bid for funding to the region, and is advised by the AIDS Working Party.

The voluntary sector has been funded by local authority and regional health authority grants, and by its own fund raising activities.

Successful bids have been made to a charity for a one-year medical post in terminal care, and a bid to the region for a terminal care team has also been successful. The latter bid had to be produced at short notice, and a small group of key people were involved. As a result of this bid, it is hoped to provide a 24-hour cover so that more people dying with AIDS can choose to have terminal care at home.

Prevention and health promotion

Those involved locally in health promotion meet regularly as the Health Promotion Sub-Group of the AIDS Liaison Group. This sub-group is chaired by the District Health Promotion Adviser, and there are representatives from the three environmental health departments, the Sussex AIDS Centre and Helpline, social services, education, the Drug Dependency Unit and the Drug Advice and Information Service (DAIS).

The Health Promotion Adviser for AIDS has undertaken a wide variety of preventive work, including an in-service programme for schools. Each secondary school was offered two sessions of training and there was a very good response to this initiative, while there was reasonable enthusiasm for the two sessions held for primary school teachers. Materials have been produced locally which are suitable for use with teenagers and with 8–11-year-olds, in conjunction with a leaflet for parents. HIV teaching has already been integrated into the schools programme, and is included in personal and social education teaching or as part of a general health education course.

Evaluation of these health promotion programmes is carried out by the health promotion adviser. A survey of schools will be undertaken to assess the value of AIDS work already undertaken.

The Health Promotion Department is also taking part in the three-year project run by Christchurch College, Canterbury, which will look into the attitudes and beliefs of school children, governors and teachers. An interim report was produced in January 1989.

Students from Brighton Polytechnic have taken part in AIDS/HIV sessions, as have staff from Brighton College of Technology and Lewes Technical College. Sussex University has its own preventive team.

Sessions have also been held with numerous groups including St John Ambulance, housing departments, refuse collectors, church groups of several denominations, Citizens' Advice Bureaux, the 'Crossroads' scheme, venture scouts, youth workers, women's groups and private nursing homes.

A voluntary helpline has long been established. The Sussex AIDS Centre and Helpline employs a full-time health education officer whose work is described in more detail later on. In addition, the Sussex AIDS Centre and Helpline and the staff development officer from the social services department are involved in the training of social services staff. The health promotion adviser from the health authority also helps social services in organising foster parents for HIV antibody-positive children.

The Drug Advice and Information Service (DAIS) is involved in preventive work, and works jointly with the Sussex AIDS Centre and Helpline to advise drug users. The drug dependency unit is involved in preventive work, and has a newly appointed full-time member of staff working specifically on HIV issues and drug use.

Local environmental health departments have concentrated on AIDS/HIV issues in the workplace, in catering and in hotel work, and have held programmes for groups of local authority staff. A seminar on HIV infection in the workplace, organised jointly by interested agencies in Brighton, was attended by 130 local employers.

There is an ongoing awareness training programme for health authority staff. HIV infection has proved to be a useful catalyst in the development of staff training. Those involved in teaching are:

- The consultant microbiologist and the infection control nurse
- The Department of Genito-urinary Medicine (consultant, health advisers, clinical nurse manager)
- The Health Promotion Department
- The Maternity Department
- The Professional Development Department
- The Occupational Health Department
- The sister in charge of in-patient care for people with AIDS

Staff groups with specific training programmes include community nurses and midwifery, paediatric and psychiatric staff. In addition, staff are granted study leave to attend appropriate courses. A programme of lectures has been held for GPs. Four AIDS and counselling workshops, lasting for two days with a follow-up study day, have been run jointly by the Health Promotion Department and the counsellor from the Department of Genito-urinary Medicine. A five-day multi-disciplinary course for trainers and supervisors has been held, and further workshops on AIDS and counselling are planned. A second series of lectures for GPs is taking place but attendance has been disappointing.

Although many staff have received some training, there has not been a

Table 12 Gonorrhoea and early infectious syphilis reports in Brighton Health Authority

	Gonorrhoea	*Early infectious syphilis*
1981	500	39
1982	480	28
1983	387	25
1984	374	28
1985	327	16
1986	289	18
1987	156	12
1988	82	6

formal training programme for all staff. A district trainer has just been designated who will be involved in setting up a full training programme.

A booklet entitled *HIV Infection and AIDS: Notes for nurses* has been produced locally to supplement in-service training. A quarterly newsletter is sent to GPs by the SCM (EH), which includes the latest AIDS and HIV figures. In the latest issue, a list of AIDS resources was distributed, together with copies of leaflets which have been produced locally.

Cases of gonorrhoea and early infectious syphilis are regularly monitored to estimate the extent to which safer sex behaviour is being adopted. It is encouraging that the numbers of cases of these two conditions have decreased significantly since 1985. This worrying trend has been observed in both young heterosexuals and young homosexuals.

Relationships with the local media have been variable. One local newspaper has a responsible attitude, and has been helpful. In others, reporting has been sensationalised.

Service provision

Primary medical care was initially provided mainly by a small number of interested and concerned GPs. However, more GPs are now involved in caring for people with HIV infection and AIDS. Volunteer organisations have not been aware of any difficulties in registration until recently, but since one of the authors of this paper has left general practice to become involved in palliative care, there have been some problems. This highlights the key role of interested and committed individuals at this stage in the epidemic.

A GP with considerable local experience has identified a number of problem areas:
- Lack of hospice provision.
- Difficulties in coping at home by people with AIDS with symptoms such as incontinence, severe diarrhoea, blindness and psychiatric symptoms.
- Feelings of helplessness and inadequacy in medical and nursing staff, and difficulties in coping with multiple bereavements.
- Prejudice and negative attitudes towards homosexuality, both in the general public and sometimes in professionals.
- Problems with the poor state of repair of the in-patient unit (now replaced).
- Concerns about HIV antibody testing.

Local authority services are provided when necessary. At first, staff such as home-helps and their managers expressed some anxiety about personal safety, but this has now been resolved. Brighton Borough Council has its own comprehensive AIDS policy, and East Sussex County Council Social Services Department published its own in January 1987.

After some initial fears were allayed, community nurses were trained to look after AIDS patients, and their care is now considered to be part of the nurses' normal work.

Most out-patient care takes place at the Genito-urinary Medicine (GUM) Clinic, although many attend with problems which could be more appropriately dealt with in primary care. Some patients who are HIV-positive and who attend the GUM clinic do not want their GPs to be informed. The GPs find this a very difficult situation, feeling that they cannot give proper care without full information. This problem is more common with asymptomatic HIV infection than with advanced AIDS.

In-patient care is provided mainly on two hospital sites. People with chest complaints are admitted to the specialised chest unit, and those with psychiatric conditions are admitted when necessary to a psychiatric unit. Other people with AIDS/HIV infection were (until spring 1987) admitted to single-room accommodation in a dilapidated ward which had traditionally been used for infectious diseases. The poor state of accommodation was the subject of considerable criticism by the patients and their advocates. As a result, the ward had to be closed, and patients were then looked after on several medical wards.

Problems with this arrangement included:

- lack of special expertise in nursing staff and concerns over personal safety.
- the loss of a particularly sympathetic, experienced and emotionally supportive nursing team which had existed in the old unit.
- pressure on medical beds which meant that arranging admissions was very time consuming.
- difficulties in the collation of information on numbers of admission, length of stay, etc. required by the AIDS Control Act.

A new six-bed in-patient ward opened in autumn 1988, funded by the regional AIDS allocation. This new ward is on the same site as chest medicine, and is intended to be of sufficient size to enable patients on zidovudine to be admitted for short stays when necessary. Out-patients are seen in the usual clinics.

Major concerns have been expressed by the Sussex AIDS Centre and Helpline about terminal care services. It has not always been possible to provide the level of round-the-clock care and support needed by a person dying at home. Despite intensive volunteer support, some people who wished to die at home have had to be admitted to an acute medical ward for terminal care. Arrangements for terminal care are being improved, however, and a charitable trust has been set up to raise funds for a hospice team.

Support for hospital staff is available through the GUM clinic, where regular sessions are held with an experienced psychologist. This support needs to be extended to other staff, and should follow when a full-time psychologist is appointed in the near future.

Where there have been confidentiality problems, they have arisen from friends and colleagues of people with HIV infection. This problem is discussed with clients during counselling pre- and post-antibody testing.

Research projects currently being undertaken by the GUM clinic include:

- Concord I international study in which asymptomatic HIV antibody-positive people will be given treatment with zidovudine and followed up over three years.

- A Medical Research Council study on heterosexual transmission of HIV infection.

- A study to assess the effectiveness of Thymopoietin III fractions (starting in February 1989).

- A PHLS study on HIV antibody prevalence in genito-urinary medicine clinic attenders.

The Sussex AIDS Centre and Helpline's response to the AIDS challenge: local issues

The first voluntary initiatives undertaken in the district were those of the gay community, at that time considered to be the only group likely to require services. This led to the setting up of the Sussex AIDS Helpline, which in three years has changed from being purely a telephone information/ counselling service operated by 7 volunteers to become an organisation numbering, at present, 120 volunteers and 7 paid staff.

For the first two years, the Helpline was funded almost entirely by its own voluntary efforts, although initial grants of £500 came from the Terrence Higgins Trust and the Family Planning Association. The first successful large-scale funding application was made to the East Sussex HIV/AIDS counselling and social work co-ordinator. This came from a recognition on the part of the social services department that, although there had been problems in the handling of the first cases, its own budgetary constraints made it difficult to create a new post internally. Another important factor in the application's success was that the then Chair of the Helpline was also an employee of the Department, and was well placed to be offered the post on the basis of his experience and contacts. The funding was made on a three-year basis.

The second major grant came from Brighton Council for the post of health education officer, and was obtained through normal voluntary organisation grant application procedures. This funding is negotiated each year, and there is always uncertainty about future funding. The third and largest grant came from the South East Thames Regional Health Authority for the current financial year, and was in large part due to a recognition of the value-for-money services provided by the Helpline and of the need to expand current staffing and office-based premises to meet current and future demands. This grant has to be negotiated each year.

The Helpline is committed to a two-pronged approach: care for those already with the infection; and education/prevention. Its policy is to care for people in their own homes, and to provide education and support in familiar surroundings. In its work, it has concentrated on individual health promotion as the best way for individuals to accept information and to effect behavioural change. One of the main functions of the Helpline to date has been to act as an 'advocate' for people with AIDS/HIV infection – e.g. directing people to the appropriate statutory agencies when there are problems of harassment. Despite its funding and its contacts with the relevant agencies, the Helpline is still able to take an independent and critical look at the care provided by the statutory authorities.

The Helpline has a responsibility for Sussex, not just Brighton, and therefore has established close links with the statutory sector by representation on various AIDS liaison groups – e.g. South East Thames Regional Health Authority and Brighton, Worthing, Hastings and Mid Downs Health Authorities. The Helpline is also in the process of establishing more informal meetings with workers in other voluntary agencies who have been identified as being HIV counsellors, health education workers or specialists within those agencies. The training given by the Helpline to other organisations has often acted as a catalyst for further initiatives. It receives referrals directly from health authority and social services staff and from other voluntary agencies, and on an individual basis. Successful liaison has been crucial to the Helpline. Although outside agencies now refer cases to the Helpline and value its work, it took time for trust to build up.

Health education, liaison and training
Links are maintained through the Health Promotion Sub-group of the AIDS Liaison Group. This tends to be a task-oriented group, to avoid duplication of work. The Helpline is paid a consultancy fee for providing a continuing training programme for East Sussex County Council social services staff. Feedback has been positive.

The use of volunteers in health promotion work
The Helpline currently employs only one full-time health education officer (HEO). In order to maximise use of this individual's time, a volunteer resourcing model has been developed. The HEO is responsible for identifying and developing projects and will liaise with all relevant agencies if necessary. It is also the HEO's responsibility to develop specific materials and approaches.

Once a programme has been piloted and evaluated, volunteers are trained in the skills necessary to continue it. The usual problem associated with the use of volunteers has been encountered – that is the uncertain availability of volunteers, who cannot guarantee long-term commitment to the programme.

The Helpline encourages male and female volunteers, irrespective of sexual preference, to work with an increasing number of antibody-positive individuals and people with AIDS. In practice, while the male/female volunteer ratio is 1:1, the majority of the males are gay men, and there is difficulty in recruiting heterosexual male volunteers.

The first phase of the Helpline programme to be developed is aimed at fifth and sixth formers, and this has been run at six secondary schools. It may seem surprising that the parental response has been so supportive, but, to some extent, they have been relieved that their children are receiving accurate information. In addition, through liaison with the YMCA drugs education project, a programme for schools has been put together.

Working with drug agencies

Drug agencies felt inadequate when dealing with HIV infection, as did the Helpline when dealing with drug problems. The development of links between the two sectors has enabled both to share information and develop confidence in other fields. Services have been developed jointly, in order to make more effective use of scarce resources.

A specific group related to drug use and HIV – the joint Sussex AIDS Centre and Helpline/Drugs Advice and Information Service (DAIS) drugs group – has been created within the Helpline to act as a forum for the sharing of inter-agency experience and for health education and support strategy development. In addition, it provides a forum for identifying and challenging prejudices held about drug use, sexual orientation and HIV generally.

The joint group is made up of representatives of the following agencies:
- Sussex AIDS Centre and Helpline
- DAIS
- the drug dependency unit
- the GUM clinic

Through this group, the Helpline (with its extensive experience of the needs of people with HIV infection) and drug agencies (with their experience of the needs of those who use drugs) aim to:
- Provide information about safer drug use and safer sex geared specifically towards drug users.
- Provide an access point to the Helpline's Body Positive and Frontliners groups for drug users who have HIV/AIDS. (The Body Positive group includes people who have asymptomatic HIV infection; Frontliners have been diagnosed as having AIDS.)

In practice, however, only a small number of drug users have so far joined Body Positive, and it remains to be seen whether other drug users will want support from the existing groups. There may be a need to set up a separate group in the future.

Once initial objectives had been identified and approved by the group, it was felt by all agencies concerned that time should be spent exploring the attitudes and beliefs of all group members to consolidate working relationships. Consequently a joint training day was organised at which members of relevant agencies brought participants up to date with new developments in their specific fields. Meetings of this kind provide a unique and vital opportunity to explore issues such as professional boundaries and territoriality to ensure that these potential obstacles are not allowed to interfere with crucial work once it has been undertaken.

There have been a number of successful projects to date.

Support for the Drug Advice and Information Service (DAIS)

A group of Helpline volunteers now hold regular counselling sessions at DAIS on risk reduction, safer sex and safer drug use. These volunteers have undergone intensive training, within both the Helpline and DAIS. This sessional input provides a valuable ongoing contact on familiar ground between the Helpline and the drug-using community, exploding such myths as 'AIDS Helplines are exclusively run by gay men for gay men.' An extremely positive outcome of this project is that drug-using individuals who were not known to either the drug dependency unit or DAIS have been presenting for information and advice at this session.

The 'Wraps' project

The 'Wraps' project (evaluated in the June edition of *Druglink*) prints information on paper squares which are of the size used to package heroin and amphetamine sulphate deals. The information includes such things as the telephone numbers of the Helpline and the Drug Advice and Information Service, and details of a sympathetic pharmacist who will provide needles. Pads of these paper squares are being distributed into drug dealer networks.

Needle exchange

Although needle exchange schemes had been discussed by the various statutory agencies, no definite action had been taken. Then the Helpline called a meeting of all those involved and, as a result, it was agreed to draw up a bid for funding. Given the wide spectrum of agencies involved in all stages of the needle exchange debate, the project is assured of extensive support from a whole series of disciplines, ranging from primary care teams to the police and the Environmental Health Department.

Analysis

Brighton has had five years of experience with HIV infection and AIDS, and the initial problems due to the inexperience of staff in statutory agencies are now in the past. Recent problems in service provision will be resolved this year by an increased level of funding.

'Ownership' of AIDS remains an issue, and there are still occasional difficulties in relationships between voluntary and statutory agencies. There are separate AIDS forums for senior hospital staff and for AIDS liaison, and there is some agenda overlap between these two groups.

At a time when there are resource constraints, separate funding for AIDS has been vital for the development of services. The voluntary sector has played a dynamic role, bringing issues to the attention of the statutory agencies and always keeping AIDS to the fore among local priorities.

In all aspects of AIDS care, both voluntary and statutory, the influence of enthusiastic and committed individuals has been substantial. AIDS has drawn together people from varying backgrounds and disciplines in a constructive way, and has provided a basis for collaborative work. There is still evidence of prejudice and ignorance, but health promotion staff and those of the voluntary agencies are working steadily to change this.

Brighton is now in the 'second phase' of its involvement with the AIDS and HIV epidemic. The first phase comprised initial staff training, development of policy and guidelines, dealing with the fears precipitated by the first few cases, and the development of inter-agency forums. There is a solid base of local health promotion work.

In the next phase, it is hoped to provide a more complete care package, including hostel care and terminal care, which can be developed to cope with the projected increase in cases.

An Integrated Response to HIV and AIDS in Oxfordshire

Dick Mayon-White, Gorm D. Kirsch and Dr Peter Anderson

The Oxfordshire Health District has a resident population of 473,942 (1981 census), which is increasing at an estimated rate of 8.9 per cent per decade. It is a relatively young population, with 66 per cent of people under 45 years of age, compared with 62 per cent in England and Wales as a whole. Oxfordshire also has a higher proportion (29 per cent) of people in social classes I and II, but the same proportion in social classes IV and V.

A first impression of Oxfordshire, with its many villages and small towns, is that it is rural. However, a closer look reveals a mixed urban/rural scene with well-established industries in the two main towns, Banbury and Oxford, and growing businesses in the market towns. There is little dense urban housing, but students and young families often live in crowded accommodation. The population is mobile, obviously because of the university and polytechnic college, and also because of developments in light industry creating skilled employment. There is a large flux of visitors, with conferences and tourists. About 2–3 per cent of people belong to ethnic minorities; there are no special religious or cultural features.

The Oxfordshire Health District is not quite coterminous with the county of Oxfordshire, because the area near Henley is served by Reading in the West Berkshire Health Authority. Oxford County Council (responsible for education and social services) and the five district councils (responsible for environmental health and housing) determine their policies in consultation with the Oxfordshire Health Authority. This is achieved by joint care-planning teams, an environmental health liaison group and collaboration between officers of the various authorities. The Health Education Unit is jointly funded by the Oxfordshire Education Department and the Oxfordshire Health Authority. There is a voluntary organisation – OXAIDS – which provides AIDS-related advice, education and care in Oxfordshire, and which is supported by grants from several agencies, including a district council, and by accommodation in the health authority's premises. Other voluntary organisations, the churches and housing associations have worked in collaboration with the health authority, but not specifically on AIDS.

The general practitioner services are administered by the Oxfordshire Family Practitioner Committee. There are 313 principal GPs. The local authorities and the health authority (since 1974) have provided health centres and community nurses for some GPs, with close links between them and health authority staff.

The Oxfordshire Health Authority is responsible for seven large hospitals (two acute general, two with a variety of specialties, two psychiatric, one orthopaedic), one small hospital for mental handicap and dermatology, and 12 community hospitals. There are also two private hospitals with links, via staff and services, to the NHS hospitals.

This is a teaching district with a wide range of regional specialties. In the context of AIDS, it provides a regional immunology service, and has the only infectious diseases specialists in the region, a regional public health laboratory and a haemophilia centre which has patients from beyond the region's boundaries. Oxford University medical school contributes heavily to the clinical and diagnostic services in the district. The Regional Health Authority, with its offices sited in the district, supports some of the university posts, notably in the Department of Community Medicine and General Practice, thus encouraging strong links between the various medical organisations.

Oxfordshire is placed in an interesting position with respect to AIDS. There is much travel to and from foreign countries, as well as commuters to London and villagers who live and work in small communities. There is a strange mixture of tolerance and bigotry, which academic life may foster.

The prevalence of infection

Patients with AIDS were treated in Oxford hospitals in 1983 (at the start of the British epidemic), but numbers have not increased quickly, and so there has been time to prepare. There is a general sense that prevention is both urgent and important because of the youth and mobility of the population. Although there were some people who said, 'It won't happen here' or 'Why all the fuss about a few cases?', such views did not obstruct the more common expression of reasonable concern.

The prevalence of HIV infection in the district is difficult to estimate because our information is drawn from clinical settings. People seek advice from the genito-urinary medicine physicians, GPs, infectious disease physicians, haematologists and psychiatrists (about drug use); all can test and counsel. To date, 68 people have been found to be infected, plus 135 patients at the supra-regional haemophilia centre. Twenty-four people have developed AIDS, of whom 14 have died.

Most risk factors have been seen: homosexual and heterosexual contacts in Britain and abroad, injecting drug use, Factor VIII injections, mother-baby transmission. Homosexuality is the most common factor among patients with AIDS, and haemophilia the most common for HIV positivity. Infection has been found in health care workers, but no occupational infection has been detected.

Approximately half of the patients with AIDS treated in Oxford live outside the district. In turn, a number of Oxford residents have gone to London, and a few have returned home to their native countries. There is a regional scheme to count cases, which preserves confidentiality by using limited coded identification. Reports have been checked against CDSC data and the counts of other districts to try to prevent double counting and to ensure complete reporting. There has been no attempt to screen samples of the population.

The response to the problem

The initial structural response was the formation of a district AIDS taskforce in 1986, with representatives of the departments and units most involved, including a health education officer, a local government liaison officer, a finance officer, a planning officer and a GP. The taskforce began as a group of ten people, selected because they were known to be interested, but its size grew as more people became involved, and eventually it became too large for practical executive functions. Therefore, a small 'mini' taskforce of six members was formed in March 1988, meeting monthly to determine the strategy of the district's AIDS work.

The mini taskforce comprises a community physician (chairman), a genito-urinary physician, an infectious disease physician, a senior nurse, a psychiatrist and a virologist. The minutes of its meetings are sent to all members of the full taskforce, and any member is welcome to attend the monthly meeting if the discussion is relevant to him/her. Tactical matters of practice and the implementation of policy are settled by individual departments, with the taskforce providing co-ordination, settlement of controversial issues and, most importantly, anticipation of forthcoming problems.

The district does not have a complete set of policies on the subject of AIDS. This is partly because the taskforce has tried to integrate the work into normal clinical practice, and partly because of a reluctance to write detailed specific policies when there was better guidance from other sources. However, we feel an increasing need for better definition of local policy and practice to respond to the pressure from staff for clear guidance on matters which have been the subject of debate. Therefore we have helped to write a regional strategy, in order to have a framework for district plans and to promote a consistency in practice with neighbouring districts. One example of this is a regional policy for health care staff who have HIV infection, which is about to be incorporated into the district policy for occupational health. Another is a workshop for the full taskforce, to review the care of patients from pre-diagnosis to death and to improve resources and co-ordination.

Funding

The funding for AIDS work has come from seven different sources, each found more by chance than by design:

(1) The substantial costs of hospital treatment of AIDS patients have been absorbed into the acute hospital budgets (and must contribute to their overspending).

(2) Small well-marked sums have been spent from the general district budget on specific items – e.g. a new bronchoscope, a share of the local government AIDS liaison officer's salary.

(3) The regional health authority has given extra support for counselling and testing in the genito-urinary departments (£50,000 in the current year).

(4) The regional health authority has funded work in prevention in three main ways: the general field of health education, developing programmes to minimise harm to injecting drug users, and enabling the appointment of the district's primary care facilitator.

(5) The Department of Health's special funds for AIDS have been allocated to programmes aimed at preventing the spread of HIV among injecting drug users.

(6) The Public Health Laboratory Service (PHLS) has given invaluable laboratory support.

(7) The regional health authority has funded regional specialities (immunology and the haemophilia centre). This includes the sum of £450,000 for heat-treated Factor VIII, which is half of the funding allocated for AIDS to the regional health authority from the Department of Health. There is conflict about whether the regional AIDS budget should be charged for the manufacture of Factor VIII, a drug not directly related to AIDS required by haemophiliacs residing outside the region.

The planning of financial support has not been easy, because the special funds from the Department of Health have come without much warning and no consultation on whether they are too much or too little. Senior managers have been more interested in other financial matters, perhaps because AIDS represents less than 1 per cent of the expenditure of the district health authority.

Health education and prevention

The work in health education and prevention in the district has ranged from that aimed at the general population to that for obvious target groups (schools, NHS staff, drug users, students). To be self-critical, our first steps in prevention were superficial because we rushed to cover too many fronts at once. We are now building up a more concentrated and stronger campaign for schools, health staff and drug users. As a result of the innovative short-term appointments of an AIDS liaison officer and a primary care facilitator (described below), we have made good progress with the colleges in Oxford, the primary care teams, community nurses and

Table 13 AIDS education activities in Oxfordshire, 1986–8

- 21 study days for workers involved with young people (including schools), with 4 additional workshops for secondary school teachers and 4 for primary school teachers, and 2 seminars for school governors.

- 20 workshops for City Council staff; 2 seminars for environmental health officers.

- 8 open lectures to hospital staff, 4 workshops for psychiatric hospital staff, 10 seminars for community health staff, and formal teaching to nurses, medical students and doctors.

- 10 seminars for social workers, child-care workers and home-helps employed by the Social Services department.

- 2 weekend courses and 15 seminars for voluntary advisers.

- 3 residential counselling courses.

- 5 one-day conferences for religious organisations.

- Training days for drug workers, prison officers, Red Cross members, student welfare officers, health and safety officers and journalists.

- 5 neighbourhood information and advice stalls during an 'AIDS awareness' week, and stalls at City Council health events.

- More than 300 individual talks and demonstrations to a wide range of audiences including youth groups; secondary school pupils, parents, governors and teachers; adult education students; further education students; university and polytechnic college students and staff; ethnic minority groups; religious groups; gay and lesbian groups; employers' associations and trade union branches; the fire service; ambulance staff; first aiders; deaf centre staff; funeral directors; opticians; pharmacists; probation officers; young offenders; hostel workers; housing associations; Housewives' Register groups; Women's Institute groups; women's health workers; rotary clubs; the Samaritans; political associations.

- The production of: leaflets for households in Oxford, for students, for the workplace and for drug-users; a minority language resource pack; a training pack for workers for people with handicaps; contributions to local bulletins, newsletters, newspapers and broadcasts; a portable poster display.

pharmacists. The drug counsellors have worked extra paid sessions to cover the county with advice, and a drugs outreach worker has started to find ways of helping drug users who have no other contact with health and voluntary services.

Our priorities for preventive work were determined by agreeing where there were gaps in our services which could be filled efficiently using local experience and knowledge. Fortunately, there were no insoluble clashes of opinion on priorities (a minor triumph of good will by Oxford's standards!). The consensus may have been easier to reach because most of the major decision-makers have been in post and working on one or more aspects of AIDS since 1983, and have shared the experience of AIDS as an increasing problem.

The AIDS liaison officer

In July 1986, the City of Oxford District Council and the Oxfordshire Health Authority appointed an AIDS liaison officer. The appointment was made jointly, with officers of both authorities writing the job description and interviewing the candidates together. This strengthened the post when the role of the liaison officer was subsequently challenged from various quarters.

The appointment received considerable publicity, mostly in support of the proposed work of this officer. This publicity proved to be a mixed blessing. It did help to get the job off to a flying start – there was no need to explain who the officer was – but more time was required to correct misunderstandings about his role (e.g. letters from school governors about teaching about 'perversions' in schools). We should have been more careful to ease the demands on the officer for him to talk about his work to audiences in other parts of the country – his work has been caught up in the 'healthy cities' movement. However, other cities have now employed their own AIDS workers.

The achievements of the Oxford AIDS liaison officer in two years have been impressive. He talked to every type of audience in the county, and was well received by most. He stimulated many local organisations to think about their policies in relation to AIDS, and arranged publicity events such as stalls at health fairs and a poster display for public places. He liaised between OXAIDS and the two employing authorities, and acted as the secretary to the AIDS liaison committee. He played a very useful role supporting the educational work of the department of genito-urinary medicine. His supervision on behalf of the health authority was given by the consultant physician in genito-urinary medicine. He had a desk in this department as well as in the environmental health department – which led to some difficulty in knowing where he was (complicated by the fact that he would be out talking, meeting or otherwise liaising most of the time). So we learned the lesson that a good office backup is essential.

It is worth stressing that this was a joint appointment, by two very different organisations – that is, the health authority and the district council. This is not an easy arrangement since both employers have their own objectives. In the second year, we developed a contract system, whereby projects were defined and agreed with specific funding by a steering group of people from both authorities. This brought more order to the demands upon the liaison officer's time, and we are planning to continue the post, perhaps with more local authorities involved and more emphasis on liaison and the training of staff than on health education.

The primary care facilitator

Another initiative started in August 1987 with a programme designed to improve the response of primary care teams to patients with HIV-related problems. We anticipated that the problems would range from the 'worried well' and people about to go on holidays abroad to people dying from AIDS at home. As with the AIDS liaison officer, there was a substantial foundation of knowledge and collaboration on which to build the new post. Work in general practice aimed at preventing heart disease and strokes had been facilitated in the county for more than four years, so the skills required to gain entry and stimulate the interest of primary health care teams were known. Arguments about the meaning and use of the word 'facilitator' had already been settled, but we had to be careful not to say 'facilitator for HIV infection' as a shortened version of 'facilitator for the prevention and care of HIV infection in general practice'. Since AIDS was still a sensitive subject, some doctors picked on such ambiguities to relieve their feelings about risk behaviour.

We were confident that training would be useful to primary care teams. In 1986, we made a telephone survey of people living in and around Oxford to find out what they knew about AIDS and where they gained their information (Hill and Mayon-White, 1987). Family doctors were one of the main sources of advice for people worried about AIDS. In the spring of 1987, we surveyed GPs in Oxfordshire and found that more than a quarter had already been involved in the care of an HIV-infected person, and that all had been consulted on the subject by patients. We learned about the areas of uncertainty in their knowledge, what they thought would be helpful, and how willing they were to look after patients with AIDS (Anderson and Mayon-White, 1988).

We also gave a series of talks to community nurses during the summer of 1987. A survey showed that they compared favourably with other professional groups in the health authority in their knowledge of HIV infection and the positive attitudes they exhibited concerning the care of people with AIDS (Klimes *et al.*, 1988). An indication of their positive attitude was their expressed wish to train with the primary care facilitator so that they would be well prepared to treat patients with AIDS at home.

Once we had decided to establish this post, we were fortunate in obtaining money for a one-year appointment from the regional health promotion fund. The job description was written with the help of the senior community nurses and other facilitators; we strongly recommend that an experienced facilitator is consulted when creating such a post.

Our Department of Community Medicine, in which the facilitator is based, had close links with GPs, practice nurses and community nurses, and a pattern of giving them information about infectious diseases was already established. The skill of the facilitator is to increase that flow of information, to ensure that it reaches all practices and is understood, and that there are no obstacles to putting the knowledge into practice. The high frequency of contacts between most people and their family doctors creates many opportunities to give advice on health matters. Immunisations for travel abroad, prescribing oral contraceptives, treating minor infections and providing medical reports for life assurance purposes can all be used for this.

It is likely that a successful facilitator will change professional attitudes, but this is not an explicit part of the job description. We hope that the interest of doctors and nurses in HIV infection and its prevention will increase as a result of having a facilitator. The facilitator can be of practical help by showing practices how they can overcome minor but important technical snags related to the management of HIV infection in the community.

The 'technical snags' are the small, often irritating difficulties that can consume a lot of time. For example, they arise with questions of clinical waste disposal, the sterilisation of equipment, the means of communication with hospital staff or social workers, the purchase of clean needles for drug users, opening times of specialist clinics, the loan of video machines for health education. The facilitator soon found what were the most common snags and how some practices had overcome them. In some cases, the solution came from feeding back questions to managers in the health authority. In a few instances, there was no direct solution – e.g. a comparison of the performances of small sterilisers and autoclaves was not published until July 1988 – but at least the facilitator could explain the position.

It is taking time to develop shared care between different medical teams. Joint meetings at which cases are reviewed have helped, and joint clinics are planned. This liaison within the hospital is essential, but the next step must be to involve the primary care teams. In the past, GPs have had difficulty in getting to case conferences on other medical and social problems. This was partly because of the length of the conferences and because they were held in central offices, a long way from most surgeries. In addition, patients with haemophilia come with most of their medical problems to the haemophilia centre, thus bypassing their family doctors, and people who have presented first at the genito-urinary medicine department also tend to remain with the specialists. So there are potential gaps if problems arise with other members of their families or when the specialist clinics are closed.

The role of the facilitator is to reduce these gaps by making the primary care teams ready to take on the care when asked. The facilitator is not privy to information about individual patients, and does not act as the intermediary between hospital and general practice in this respect. As it is, the facilitator is fully occupied without individual casework. Ideally, we should like to avoid the need for 'key workers' for patients, because patients with their relations and close friends should be able to control their own care. Our patients with HIV infection have not been socially isolated – in fact, in some cases there seem to be almost too many people waiting to advise and support. We recognise that this state may change as numbers increase. The primary care teams must be ready for patients who do not wish, for various reasons, to follow the standard patterns of care.

The pay and conditions of service of the facilitator are equivalent to those of a community nursing sister or health visitor. Our facilitator had experience of nursing AIDS patients at home, which has been very useful in training community nurses. A willingness to travel has also been an asset appreciated by the primary care teams who are visited by the facilitator in their own premises. Contrary to popular expectations, the patients with AIDS have not been concentrated in the city; rather, their homes are in the villages and small market towns where four-fifths of Oxfordshire's people live. As a result, 'distance learning' is required. The facilitator produces a regular bulletin, with features on the medical aspects of the HIV-related diseases, items of news, tips on good practice, and references to sources of further information.

The facilitator post has been enough of a success for neighbouring districts to wish to join in the scheme. The informal feedback from practices in the district has been favourable. We can see that practices are being visited and that information is being exchanged. We do not yet know if this is beneficial to patients or whether it will be. We have thought carefully about how one could evaluate the efficacy of the work, but the problem is that changes are happening so quickly that a before-and-after survey would be misleading. A controlled trial is needed to compare practices that have been visited by a facilitator with those that have not, but we have few unvisited practices in our district.

Haemophilia

Oxford has a centre which treats about 300 haemophiliac patients from within and without the region. Of these, 135 patients are HIV antibody-positive, and 9 have had AIDS. It has been more straightforward to arrange care and treatment for these patients than might have been expected from the accounts of AIDS in other cities. This has probably less to do with attitudes towards the means whereby they became infected than to the fact that they were already patients and clients. Once a caring relationship is established, it is not easily broken by irrational fears of infection, so medical treatment and social support have continued without interruption and with the minimum of fuss.

It has been possible to discuss patients' problems a little more openly because of this constructive atmosphere, but there have been at least two distressing episodes when information was spread too widely. Haemophilia patients with HIV or AIDS are as sensitive and vulnerable to ostracism as people exposed to the infection in other ways. Therefore we try to apply the formula of 'only those who need to know' when arranging support at home or school.

Patients with haemophilia and their friends and families are not a completely distinct 'risk group'. For many, the injection of blood product and a monogamous sexual relationship are the only risk factors, but some are injecting drug users and some have had more than one sexual partner. They are one of the most carefully and regularly counselled groups, so further transmission from them would be an important indication of the efficacy of counselling.

We noted above that family doctors may not be closely involved in this counselling and care, but there may be patients who will feel antagonistic towards the place that has given them infected Factor VIII. Relatives may feel this even more strongly than the patients, and these feelings may increase as asymptomatic infections progress to AIDS and death. Then the long distances that patients travel to the haemophilia centre may seem unbearably burdensome, and other districts may experience a sudden increase in caseloads.

The establishment of new care and counselling facilities at the haemophilia centre was managed independently of district health authority plans because extra funds from central government were allocated for this specific use. The presence of a regional or supra-regional specialist centre in a district could cause complications but, happily, this has not been a serious problem in this case. Four factors may have helped: the additional funding for haemophilia was followed by other forms of 'AIDS money' which prevented other services falling too far behind; the haemophilia centre is located close to the infectious diseases ward where patients with AIDS are cared for; the medical and nursing staff of the haemophilia centre contribute to the work of district and regional committees; and individual departmental interests are respected. It is worth noting that there have been no complaints arising from haemophilia patients being nursed on the same ward as ex-drug users or gay men.

The university

Oxford University and the other institutions of further education in the city have had an important influence on the interest in HIV infection in the district. By building on the interest shown by the students and staff, it has been possible to turn scientific curiosity about a new viral infection with wide social implications into general support for preventive work in this field.

The experience of medical clinics in the colleges and the hospitals has been that students are at risk of acquiring sexually transmitted diseases but no more so than other groups of young people. Although there are the occasional sensational accounts of student sexuality, the main impression given by formal surveys is that, for most students, sexual experiences are infrequent and limited to a small number of partners. While the prevalence of HIV infection remains low, there may be some justification for students believing that AIDS could not occur among their circle of friends. However, students tend to travel widely, and the colleges and language schools teach people from many countries, so the present, apparently low local prevalence is not much of a safeguard.

Heterosexual intercourse without contraception is not uncommon in the student population and is perhaps a reflection of limited sexual experience (Turner *et al.*, 1988). Along with the need to prevent unwanted pregnancies, the importance of promoting the avoidance of sexually transmitted infection has also been recognised. Fortunately, the college authorities have understood these needs and have granted access to health education. This co-operation had been helped by the local voluntary organisation, OXAIDS, which began health education about HIV infection in the university. The AIDS liaison officer has collaborated with OXAIDS in continuing this work. Access is facilitated by volunteers who are members of the particular university or polytechnic. Some of the requests for educational intervention also come from students who want to be active in preventing the spread of HIV infection and AIDS. Each year brings a new round of requests, which reminds us that each year there is a fresh group who need advice.

Conclusions

In this district, we are fortunate to have excellent primary care services, and experience of good co-operation between different organisations. We have tried to use the time before the expected wave of AIDS cases to strengthen existing services and to press the need for, and value of, prevention. It is likely that we have made mistakes, but we hope that we shall have put AIDS into the midst of normal medical care and not let it become a disease to be treated in isolation.

References

Anderson, P. and Mayon-White, R. T. (1988) General practitioners and the management of infection with HIV. *British Medical Journal*, 296, 535–7.

Hill, A. and Mayon-White, R. T. (1987) A telephone survey to evaluate an AIDS leaflet campaign. *Health Education Journal*, 46, 127–9.

Klimes, I., Catalan J., Bond, A. *et al.* (1988) Knowledge and attitudes of health care staff to HIV infection. Paper presented at the International Conference on AIDS, Stockholm, 1988.

Turner, C., Anderson P., FitzPatrick R. *et al.* (1988) Sexual behaviour, contraceptive practice and knowledge of AIDS in Oxford University students. *Journal of Biosocial Science*, 20, 445–51.

A Public Health Response: The experience of Bradford

Dr Kathie Marfell and June C. Whitham

On the bookcase in the office of the Medical Officer for Environmental Health in Bradford stands a card bearing these words:

O Lord, give me the serenity to accept the things I cannot change, the courage to change the things I can, and the wisdom to know the difference.

This guiding prayer seems to be ideal for a community physician committed to improving the health of one's population. Change is, however, particularly hard to achieve from the position of the 'medical officer for environmental health' or 'proper officer' or whatever the title will be following the deliberations on the Acheson Report (DHSS, 1988).

Unlike the pre-1974 medical officer of health, the medical officer for environmental health (MOEH) has no power base, no staff to manage, no budget. She has roles clearly defined in statute but no other strings to pull. She has to work through others, with officers of the local authority to whom she acts as adviser but with whom she has no managerial relationship. Most of us learn to cope with this potentially difficult working situation by making the most of what opportunities present themselves, and trying to create the opportunities we would wish to occur.

Bradford: An overview

Bradford Metropolitan District is the area administered by Bradford Metropolitan District Council (MDC). It covers an area of approximately 37,100 hectares (568 sq. km) in West Yorkshire and serves a population of 454,198 people (1981 census). The district is served by two health authorities. Bradford Health Authority (population approximately 340,000) covers the larger part of the district and is based upon the urban centres of Bradford and Shipley. Airedale Health Authority serves a population of 175,000, the majority of whom live around the urban centre of Keighley which lies within the Bradford Metropolitan District. Airedale Health Authority also covers the (much larger geographically) district of Craven in North Yorkshire, a rural area which includes the city of Skipton (Fig. 10).

Prior to the 1982 reorganisation of the National Health Service, both

Figure 10 **Bradford Metropolitan District topography and settlement**

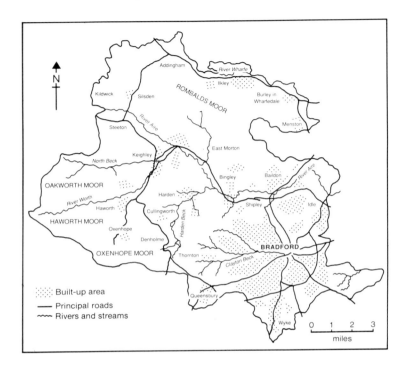

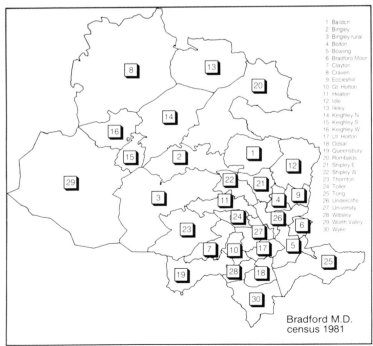

1 Baildon
2 Bingley
3 Bingley rural
4 Bolton
5 Bowling
6 Bradford Moor
7 Clayton
8 Craven
9 Eccleshill
10 Gt Horton
11 Heaton
12 Idle
13 Ilkley
14 Keighley N
15 Keighley S
16 Keighley W
17 Ltl Horton
18 Odsal
19 Queensbury
20 Rombalds
21 Shipley E
22 Shipley W
23 Thornton
24 Toller
25 Tong
26 Undercliffe
27 University
28 Wibsley
29 Worth Valley
30 Wyke

Bradford M.D.
census 1981

health districts were part of the Bradford Area Health Authority, and close links persist. Before 1982, the Area Health Authority provided a specialist in community medicine to function as medical adviser to the Bradford MDC in the role of MOEH. This arrangement has been retained, with medical advice to the MDC provided by a single doctor and the appropriate reimbursement made by Airedale Health Authority to Bradford Health Authority for this service.

This makes liaison between health and local authorities considerably easier: the MOEH has only one local authority to work with and the MDC has only one MOEH to consult. This considerably simplifies and strengthens working relationships between the two authorities, the geographical boundaries of the MOEH's responsibility being coterminous with those of the local authority.

The city of Bradford includes a university of nearly 5,000 undergraduate and postgraduate students, many of whom come from overseas (including central Africa) for its professional and technical courses. Collaborative links between the university and Bradford Health Authority were strengthened by the establishment of the Clinical Epidemiology Research Unit in 1985. This is headed by a director who is a Fellow of the Faculty of Community Medicine. He is also the district general manager of the Bradford Health Authority, and holds a personal chair in public health at the university. At the time of writing, the Bradford Health Authority has a 'post-Acheson' department of public health headed by a director of public health (previously the district medical officer) and has just published its third new-style annual report on the health of Bradford (Bradford Health Authority, 1988).

Since the 1982 reorganisation of the National Health Service, Bradford has been actively developing its public health functions by close collaboration between health and local authorities. A major epidemic of bacterial dysentery in 1984 throughout the Bradford Metropolitan District (Bandaranayake, 1985) brought together formally officers of the local authority and the two health authorities in a collaborative effort to bring the epidemic under control. Following the resolution of this particular problem, the then MOEH presented a report on the management of the outbreak to both the Bradford Health Authority and the local authority's Environmental Health Subcommittee. The health authority's response to this was to request a further report on collaboration between the two authorities.

What the health authority wanted were a few pages of commentary on how liaison operated between the two bodies. What they received was the first annual report on the health of Bradford to be produced since the demise of the post of medical officer of health.

There are many who had been glad to see the end of the old annual reports, having spent a large part of the working year in collating and presenting the statistics and writing the text. However, one of the authors of this article had wanted to raise the annual report, like a 'phoenix from the ashes', not as a predictable annual compilation of workload statistics but to serve two functions: as a reference document to compare the health of Bradfordians to their peers elsewhere in the United Kingdom; and also, and more importantly, as an agenda-setting tool to direct the attention of decision-makers in both health and local authorities to the health issues in the district.

The 1985 annual report, published in the summer of 1986, was widely read within the local authority. It was received by several groups and committees and increased the awareness of health issues by the policy makers. It also achieved wide media coverage in local newspapers and on local radio.

The AIDS Control Forum

One small paragraph in that report sparked off the public health response to AIDS in Bradford. The paragraph in question quoted national statistics only and gave local telephone numbers where advice and counselling about HIV infection could be obtained. This brief mention resulted in two columns in the local paper which quoted the MOEH. In response to that article, many local groups and individuals interested in AIDS prevention contacted the MOEH directly. Thus informal networks of interested people were created.

The now renamed Public Health and Protection Subcommittee of the local authority asked for more information about AIDS, and, in November 1986, the MOEH duly presented a paper, supported by the video produced by the Leicester Health Promotion Unit. The committee proposed the setting up of an advisory group – the AIDS Control Forum – to advise the local authority on prevention of the spread of HIV.

The next step was to obtain a budget, and the process we used was analogous to that for any outbreak or epidemic situation. Learning from our experience of managing the dysentery outbreak, particularly the need to make quick decisions about allocation of resources, we presented a report to the local authority's management team, and asked for a budget to control the HIV epidemic. This was to be controlled by the Director of Housing and Environmental Health Services, together with political leaders on the advice of the officers. At this time, an AIDS co-ordinator was appointed within the Environmental Health Department to administer the AIDS Control Forum and the initiatives arising from it.

The management team recognised the importance of the local authority in the control of communicable disease both in statute and by the nature of its work. The officers of the local authority have contact with large numbers of the general public every day. Educating local authority personnel about

AIDS would, directly and indirectly, inform a large proportion of the population of the city. We were also in a position to learn from the experience of the United States and London, and to establish prevention programmes before the emergence of our first local cases of AIDS.

These things were happening at a time of increasing public awareness of AIDS and growing governmental concern. This made local politicians very receptive to information about AIDS and keen to support local initiatives. It also meant a good attendance at the inaugural meeting of the AIDS Control Forum (a list of those invited to attend the first and subsequent meetings is given in Table 14). Perhaps surprisingly, high attendance rates have been sustained over the ensuing two years. This has been due, at least in part, to the ownership all members feel for the Forum. It is chaired by a politician (the current chair of the Public Health and Protection Subcommittee), with the health and local authority officers, as members of the Forum, on an equal footing with trade union leaders, social workers,

Table 14 **Members of the Bradford AIDS Control Forum**

- Chair (elected): current chairperson of the Public Health Subcommittee
- Opposition party AIDS spokesperson
- One representative from each directorate of the local authority
- Medical Officer for Environmental Health
- Specialist in Community Medicine (Airedale Health Authority)
- Administrator, Family Practitioner Committee
- Secretary, Local Medical Committee
- Secretary, Local Dental Committee
- Secretaries to local trade unions – e.g. NUT, NALGO, etc.
- Nursing officer responsible for family planning
- Health promotion officers
- Representative from Community Relations Council
- Representative from Community Health Council
- Superintendent, West Yorkshire Metropolitan Police
- Representative from the BRIDGE (Bradford Independent Drug Guidance and Education) Project
- Representative from Pennine AIDS Link
- Representative from Bradford Gay Switchboard Collective
- Representative from Bradford University Students' Union

voluntary workers and so on. All ideas, contributions and opinions are given equal respect by the Forum, and information on the progress of initiatives is fed back at all meetings. As a means of encouraging the less vocal majority to express their views, questionnaires have been used so that ideas can be put forward anonymously. At the time of writing, a series of workshops is being planned for the same purpose.

The local media have taken great interest in the work of the Forum and frequently report on the progress of its initiatives. These projects are always attributed to the Forum as a whole, so all members can take a pride in their joint achievements.

Health education and training

One of the early initiatives of the AIDS Control Forum concerned education and training. It was seen as important that accurate information about HIV infection should be disseminated as widely as possible. In the health authority at that time we were inundated from many quarters with requests for talks about AIDS, and the few members of staff capable of meeting this need were unable to cope with the scale of the demand. It was felt by the Forum that the only mechanism by which this expressed need could be met was by a 'cascade' training approach – that is, for a core group of about a dozen individuals to undertake the training of key personnel in health and local authorities and other relevant organisations who, in their turn, would 'train' others.

Accordingly, the core group met in February 1987 and set about planning materials and methods. This approach met with mixed success. In some areas, where the core trainer was enthusiastic and committed and his/her expertise and credentials accepted, the cascade programme was very successful. It worked particularly well in Bradford in the Directorate of Education, for example. In other areas, where the trainer was unsure and his/her credibility questioned, the cascade failed.

Learning from this experience, the response of the local authority was to appoint a team of HIV/AIDS trainers whose function would be to inform the entire staff of the local authority (some 27,000 persons) about HIV infection, the issues it raises, and the way it would affect their particular working practices. This response, of course, covers directly only the employees of Bradford MDC and meets the needs of the general public only indirectly. The needs of local groups and organisations for information continue to be met by the health authority's Health Promotion Unit.

A post of education adviser (HIV/AIDS) was also funded to advise teachers and school governors on HIV infection and its role in the syllabus. She works closely with the advisers for health education and drugs in this context.

Information for the general public has also been disseminated by two other means: the AIDS Media Panel and the AIDS Roadshow.

The Media Panel

The Media Panel was established by the AIDS Control Forum to be pro-active in getting the facts about AIDS across to the press, radio and television and thereby reduce, as far as possible, the alarmist and often irresponsible media coverage which had taken place elsewhere. The Media Panel comprises the MOEH, the senior health promotion officer who has special responsibility for AIDS, representatives from the environmental health and social services departments of the local authority and also from Pennine AIDS Link, a local voluntary group.

This approach has generally been successful. Among its 'coups' have been a local television news magazine 'special' during the week of the DHSS leaflet drop in which a panel of local experts answered questions posed by viewers (the panel mostly consisting of the Bradford Media Panel), and a special 'AIDS supplement' to the city's newspaper in April 1987. More important, though, was the identification of a number of people who can answer the queries of local journalists accurately and responsibly, and can offer a local angle on national news items about HIV and AIDS.

The AIDS Roadshow

The AIDS Roadshow is a truly collaborative venture. Financed via joint funding arrangements by both Bradford Health Authority and Bradford MDC, it comprises a set of Marler–Hayley panels with posters, leaflets, etc. and a van to transport them from one venue to another. It is taken out to pubs, clubs, university and colleges on request and is staffed by volunteers from Pennine AIDS Link who answer questions, distribute condoms and direct inquirers to appropriate services.

Practical measures

The other main area of interest of the Forum concerned facilitation of the health promotion messages regarding HIV infection. Two principal areas came under focus: the provision of clean equipment for drug users, and the wider availability of condoms. Sub-groups of the AIDS Control Forum were established to examine these issues in more detail and put forward a strategy to the Forum.

The needle exchange scheme

The sub-group looking at drug use comprised the MOEH, a senior counsellor from the street drug agency BRIDGE (Bradford Independent Drug Guidance and Education), a senior environmental health officer responsible for communicable disease control, a representative from Pennine AIDS Link and the secretary of the local pharmaceutical committee. The latter was included at his own suggestion as he felt that community pharmacists could be a useful resource in this context.

From discussions held by this small group, a scheme evolved for used injecting equipment to be exchanged for new replacements, based at chemists' shops. The pharmacists' representative felt confident that, since pharmacists could legally sell needles to drug users, they would be prepared to operate an exchange system whereby used equipment could be disposed of safely.

At this time, the DHSS was looking for districts to operate pilot needle exchange schemes which would concentrate on offering a counselling service to drug users, with needle exchange offered as an enticement to encourage users to come forward. In Bradford, we felt that this was not a sufficiently immediate response to the pressing need to prevent the further spread of HIV infection in this key group. Although the BRIDGE project was offered one of the DHSS pilot schemes, the offer was rejected in favour of a scheme that was acceptable and accessible to the users themselves, offered anonymity to clients and had no 'strings' attached.

The operational details of the Bradford scheme are described fully in a locally produced booklet, available from the authors of this chapter.

Availability of condoms

A second sub-group looked in detail at ways of making condoms more easily available to those at risk of HIV infection. For a number of reasons this is a much more complex issue than that of providing clean needles to drug users: the relative and not absolute protection conferred by condom usage; the need to ensure that condoms are used properly; and the difficulties inherent in reaching those individuals most 'at risk' of acquiring HIV infection sexually. We included the nursing officer responsible for family planning in this group because of her knowledge and experience in this area.

Many options were considered including free distribution through family planning clinics (rejected because of the need to differentiate between contraception and control of infection), and free distribution to the unemployed and low-waged (rejected because of administrative difficulties and potential stigmatisation of these groups). Free condoms are supplied for distribution after counselling by the authority's AIDS counsellors and by the counsellors at the BRIDGE project. Youth workers in the Youth and Community Service keep a supply of condoms for sale at subsidised cost to young people at risk, after appropriate counselling. In addition, free condoms are distributed by the AIDS Roadshow.

In addition over 50 condom vending machines have been installed in local authority buildings including offices, training centres, works depots and family centres (previously day nurseries).

The Asian community in Bradford

A particular area of local concern has been that of making information about HIV infection available to people whose first language is not English. The distinctive demographic feature of Bradford is its large population of ethnic minorities originating from southern Asia. The largest group are Muslims from the Mirpur district of Pakistan. There are, in addition, small communities of Hindus from Gujerat, Sikhs from the Punjab, East African Asians and Bengalis from the Sylhet district of Bangladesh, the latter now settled mainly in Keighley (Ballard, 1985).

The Asian community in Bradford experiences high fertility rates – 168 per 1,000 for Bradford Asians in 1985 compared with 68 for Bradford non-Asians, 63 for Yorkshire region and 61 for England and Wales (Bradford Health Authority; unpublished data). As a result, the Asian population distribution in Bradford is skewed towards the younger age groups (Fig. 11). Thus 52.6 per cent of our Asian population is under 20 years of age and only 1.1 per cent is over 65. The corresponding proportions in the non-Asian population are 31.3 per cent and 14.0 per cent.

The total Asian population in Bradford includes some 45,000 people,

Figure 11 **Age structure of the Bradford Metropolitan District population**

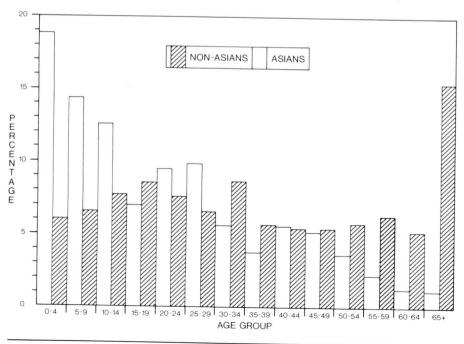

roughly 1 in 10 of the population of the Bradford Metropolitan District. A number of southern Asian languages are spoken. The Community Relations Council (CRC) in Bradford estimate the breakdown of the major languages spoken to be as shown in Table 15.

Table 15 **Major Asian languages spoken in Bradford**

Language	Population
Urdu	30,000
Punjabi	5,000
Gujerati	5,000
Bengali	3,000
Hindi	2,000

Source: Bradford Community Relations Council

In order to understand the issues surrounding AIDS and HIV infection, one has first to confront the issues surrounding sex and sexuality. The cultural traditions of the Asian population in Bradford do not encourage open discussion of these. Although the Community Relations Council has been diligent in sending a representative to the AIDS Control Forum, they have been wary of taking up the AIDS banner within their own communities and have resisted translating available English materials into Asian languages – sometimes with good reason, as these materials are culturally unsuitable in many instances.

Many exciting developments have been taking place in Bradford recently in the area of ethnic minorities' health. A health initiative funded by the DHSS is being operated through the Community Relations Council, and two workers employed in this project have attended the AIDS Control Forum.

The Bradford Health Authority was one of a number which took part in the centrally funded Asian Mother and Baby Campaign recently. As part of that campaign, we employed a number of Asian women as linkworkers to act as advocates for Asian mothers and mothers-to-be in their contacts with the NHS. After the campaign ended, the health authority continued the contracts of these women (now known as liaison officers) and indeed extended this service.

With the experience gained from this and similar ventures, and after consultation with relevant local individuals and organisations, it was agreed that the optimum approach would be a community project under the umbrella of adult and family health, within which AIDS awareness and knowledge, and understanding about HIV infection, could be explored. A project has been conceived jointly by Bradford Health Authority and Bradford MDC, together with the Health Education Authority and the Community Projects Foundation (CPF), to achieve this aim.

The Bradford Community Health Initiative

The project aims to reach out to ethnic minority groups in Bradford's communities in order to increase levels of information and knowledge about health. A community development approach will be used, linking with and working alongside existing organisations and informal networks.

The aim is to test the viability of a community development approach in communicating about health issues to local people, many of whom, because of the language and methods being used at present, are being denied opportunities to become fully informed. This applies particularly to areas of health information which are linked to cultural taboos such as drug usage, sexuality and sexually transmitted disease – including HIV infection. By working in ways which are acceptable to the cultures and traditions of the communities within our population, we hope that levels of knowledge and understanding can be increased, and that, as a result, a range of service provision will be more sensitive to the cultural needs of the community.

A project leader has been appointed to undertake the development phase which consists of discussion with organisations and groups in the city about the detailed structure of the project and where areas of work should be focused. The person appointed is recognised as 'belonging' to the Bradford Asian community, and she is already familiar with many existing community groups, having previously worked with the Community Relations Council.

Following the development phase of this initiative (probably between six and nine months), the project leader will be responsible for designing and building up of the core team, which will consist of herself and three field workers. In addition, some existing health authority staff (health promotion officers) will be linked to the project.

The Community Projects Foundation will manage the project from its Leeds office, which will also function as the liaison point for collaboration with the Health Education Authority and for evaluation and the dissemination of information. A local management committee accountable to CPF will also be established to include members of the core team and drawing upon representatives of relevant local organisations.

The project will be funded for an initial term of three years following the development phase. Evaluation and review will determine its continuation after that period. Evaluation of the project will be undertaken on a continuous basis and reported to both the Community Projects Foundation and the Health Education Authority.

Conclusion

The existing intra- and inter-organisational structures in Bradford have facilitated the individual public health responses by this city to the challenge of HIV infection. The collaboration of health and local authorities with the university and local voluntary organisations and groups has fostered and supported a peculiarly individual approach to AIDS prevention. We make no claims to having developed the right packages or 'ideal' responses – only to having done what seemed right at the time, for Bradford's communities, in response to the AIDS pandemic.

We thank all members of the AIDS Control Forum for their past efforts and continued support for the prevention of the spread of HIV in our city, and look forward to a successful collaborative venture with the Health Education Authority and the Community Projects Foundation.

References

Ballard, R. (1985). *The Ethnic Minorities in Bradford: An analysis of the 1981 census.* Applied Anthropology Group, Department of Psychology, University of Leeds.

Bandaranayake, R. (1985). The 'Bloody-Flux' – An epidemic of bacillary dysentery. In: *Case Studies in Environmental Health*, Occasional Paper No. 7. Unit for Continuing Education, Department of Community Medicine, University of Manchester.

Bradford Health Authority. (1988). *The Health of Bradford 1987.*

DHSS. (1988). *Public Health in England: The Report of the Committee of Inquiry into the future development of the public health function* (Acheson Report). London, HMSO.

Preparations for Change in North West Hertfordshire

Christopher Hayes and Dr Anne Wright

North West Hertfordshire Health Authority is situated some 30 miles north of London. There are two main centres of population at St Albans and Hemel Hempstead, and the surrounding area is essentially rural. There is some light industry, but many of the residents are employed in London. The district is generally recognised as an affluent part of England.

The health authority spans two district councils which are responsible for environmental health and housing; Hertfordshire County Council is responsible for social services and education. As in most areas, there are a great number of voluntary organisations, many of which are health related. However, until recently there was little activity in the voluntary sector concerning HIV/AIDS.

District AIDS policy

In 1986, the District Management Board of the North West Hertfordshire Health Authority established its AIDS Action Group, to co-ordinate local services, to complement the national objectives of the prevention of the spread of HIV infection, to ensure the provision of diagnostic services and to promote a better understanding of the infection. Membership is now multi-disciplinary and multi-agency, and is now chaired by the district medical officer. The group meets bi-monthly to review progress and make further recommendations as necessary.

One of the main tasks has been the production of a district strategy and a manual for health promotion, which includes the services concerned with HIV infection and AIDS. The strategy has been widely circulated and is in the process of being implemented.

Prevalence of HIV and AIDS

The number of people resident in the district both with AIDS and who have died from AIDS is very low (fewer than 10). The number who have been tested and found to be HIV-positive in the clinic in the district is equally low. The figure may be an underestimate of the true prevalence of infection because people prefer to be tested away from their area of residence and some testing centres in London are easily accessible. Informal sources suggest that many more people in the district are HIV-positive.

The prevalence of people with AIDS is monitored not only by the Communicable Disease Surveillance Centre (CDSC) but also by a confidential register maintained by the district medical officer. This has been necessary because funding from the Regional Health Authority is allocated according to the number of patients cared for in the district. The data collated by CDSC reflect only the location of the doctor submitting the report, not the area of residence where the person with AIDS is likely to require care services and support.

Health promotion and the HIV-AIDS team

The health authority's Health Promotion Unit (HPU) is located within the Department of Community Medicine at District Headquarters, and the HIV/AIDS team is part of this unit. The district health promotion officer is the co-ordinator of the HIV/AIDS programme. The team consists of five other members of staff:

- Training officer
- Volunteer co-ordinator/counsellor
- Youth and community worker
- Health promotion officer (HIV/AIDS)
- Clerical officer

The HIV/AIDS team operates in the areas of planning, staff training for the Health Service and other organisations, youth and community work, sex education in schools, volunteer co-ordination and counselling services, and community development projects. Limited secretarial support is provided, as is a computer-assisted graphic design service for the production of teaching materials, training aids, displays and publications. The team produces a bi-monthly HIV/AIDS newsletter, which is widely distributed within the health district. The team works closely with those from neighbouring health authorities.

The health authority has established an HIV/AIDS information and drop-in centre called 'The Crescent'. This centre is staffed by volunteers for whom a comprehensive selection and training programme has been provided. A Body Positive group for people with HIV infection and a 'Buddy' group to befriend and support people with AIDS have both been established.

Training

Workshops and training sessions have been offered for all health authority, education and social services staff. It is now mandatory for all health care workers employed by the authority to attend an annual in-service training session.

There has generally been good response to all the education and training programmes for staff. However, with a low reported prevalence of HIV infection, there is a problem with maintaining enthusiasm and avoiding complacency.

Service provision

People who are HIV-positive or have AIDS and require hospital admission are cared for in the general wards. While the number of these people in hospital remains low, it is sometimes difficult to preserve confidentiality. They are seen as 'special' and therefore worthy of discussion between colleagues. However, the importance of confidentiality is constantly stressed to all health care workers.

Drugs and AIDS

About 20 injecting drug users are known to local drug agencies. As it is generally accepted that only about 10 per cent are known to agencies, it can be estimated that there are probably about 200 injecting drug users in the district. Funding became available from the DHSS following the guidance set out in the circular entitled *Curbing the spread of HIV and AIDS infection* (HC[87]8). A survey and review were carried out between October 1987 and April 1988 concerning local services as well as local pharmacists' views and their willingness to become involved in a needle exchange scheme. Over 32 per cent of pharmacists are prepared to participate in such a scheme, and one is now being established, based on local pharmacies, accident and emergency departments and voluntary drug agencies. This will be supported by a health promotion officer.

Mental Handicap Unit

The North West Hertfordshire Health Authority is unique in Britain in having responsibility for three large residential mental handicap hospitals. In 1988, these three hospitals housed a total of 2,300 residents coming mainly from North West Thames Regional Health Authority; there are only 200 people with mental handicap resident in hospitals elsewhere in the Region.

As part of an overall district strategy for the control of HIV infection, the North West Hertfordshire Mental Handicap Working Party on HIV infection was convened in late 1987. This group identified general areas of need pertaining to staff and residents. These included education and training for staff and education about HIV infection (including sex education) for residents. The working party recommended that a sub-group be set up to investigate and implement a health education programme with the hospital residents on the risks and prevention of HIV infection and AIDS, for which funding has now been identified.

Background to the study

Responsibility for residents with a mental handicap lies with senior staff (nursing and non-nursing) and medical consultants. Strong emphasis is placed on developing social skills. Some patients have counselling from psychologists who do not try to influence sexual orientation – 'If they are gay, that's OK.' Staff are particularly helpful and all seem open minded and support the residents' rights to express themselves sexually.

We decided to interview a cross section of residents to ascertain the level of educational need. Meetings were arranged with the senior consultant and the senior nurse for two of the units in one hospital to discuss the project and gain their support.

Criteria for the selection of residents were extremely difficult, as we had to take into account their medical conditions, whether they were sexually active or not, levels of comprehension and verbal communication skills. In the end, residents were chosen who were known to have established relationships. Attempts were made to identify practising homosexuals in established relationships but we were not able to identify any from within this particular setting who were willing to talk to us. It was also hoped to interview residents from the community but this subsequently proved impractical in the available time scale.

From the start, it was decided that there would be no pressure on residents to take part in the project. It was felt very strongly that they should have control of their contributions.

Having identified the residents for the survey, it was arranged for the district medical officer and the district health promotion officer to meet the residents and some of the staff, so that the project could be explained to them and to seek their participation. It was stressed that we would be asking them questions concerning their knowledge and attitudes to HIV/AIDS, their sexuality and sexual experience. As might be expected, it took both the residents and the interviewers some time to get to know one other. Of the eight residents invited, five agreed to take part in the project. Between the initial meeting and the interviews, those taking part were encouraged to think about the issues and to discuss the project with their care staff and friends, and to consider its implications to themselves, retaining the option to back out if they so wished.

The interviews were taped as a means of obtaining an accurate record, permission having been sought from the residents prior to recording. Some of them afterwards enjoyed hearing themselves on tape for the first time! It was agreed that, where residents were escorted by a member of staff, it would be acceptable for him or her to sit in as a silent observer and supporter.

A structured interview pro forma was devised in order to maintain consistency in the interview techniques. The main points considered were each resident's past and present sexual history and practices, attitudes towards sex and knowledge of HIV and AIDS. In order to maintain confidentiality, it was agreed with the medical and nursing staff and the residents concerned to use pseudonyms, so they could not be identified.

The following case histories are based on interviews with the residents. They have not been validated with the care staff, except where indicated.

Case histories
Sara

Sara is 35 years old and for the last 13 years has been resident in hospital. She lives on an open single-sex ward. She claims her original admission was for teenage pregnancy and having sex with many partners for cash or other favours. Sara is a friendly, talkative person and hopes to be leaving the hospital soon and move into a hostel in Watford.

Sara has had a stable sexual partner, John, for the last eight years. He lives in a hostel outside the hospital. While Sara is monogamous, John has other girlfriends, but claims he does not have sex with them. There are no facilities in the hospital for couples to have sex. They find private places within the grounds – behind the cricket pavilion, in the bushes, behind the nurses' home or at the top of an internal fire escape. Sara visits her family for the weekend four times a year, and John has also visited with her. They have only had sex when her parents were out of the house and they were alone. Sara also visits John at the hostel. Sara is aware of contraception and some of the methods available. She has been on the contraceptive pill since 1975.

Several of Sara's early sexual partners used condoms with varying degrees of success. When Sara was asked if she had used a condom, she replied, 'Don't be silly. I haven't got a willy!' She knew that condoms were available for purchase from the hospital shop and that they cost 59p for a packet of three. Sara's weekly income is £4.50. If they were more readily available, she would prefer to get them from the hospital social club.

When asked what arrangements she would like the hospital to provide for privacy and sexual contact, her preference was for a bedroom away from the ward and ward staff.

Sara is aware of AIDS from the television, but had not discussed this with staff until just before the interviews. She is concerned about the weight loss and the 'blood test', which she associated with routine cervical smear testing. She also told us that she had heard on the radio that tablets are available to 'stop it'. She is aware that HIV/AIDS is associated with homosexual sex, but is not clear on the sex practice or the method of transmission.

Janet

Janet is 51 years old and for the last 36 years has been a resident in hospital. She lives in a single-sex villa with five other residents. With the other house members, she works on a rota for normal household chores. Janet also works in the hospital laundry for £8.00 a week and is awaiting a rise!

Janet was admitted when she was 16, following three pregnancies; she has had a total of five pregnancies resulting in two live children. Janet has had several boyfriends but now has a steady relationship with George, although she claims not to have had sex with him. She says she has had many sexual partners – residents, patients and people from outside the hospital – for cash or cigarettes.

Her view now is that sex is disgusting and that men 'get you into trouble and leave you'. When Janet has been on 'town parole,' she has been attacked twice, when men have 'taken my body'. She associates the act of sex with standing up. Janet would like to be able to have a sex partner in the villa, but would have to get permission from the staff and doctors. She has been told that, if she wants to have sex, she must 'do it outside'!

Janet is aware of contraception; she has been on the pill and now has a coil fitted. She is aware that condoms are available from the hospital shop and has seen used condoms around the hospital grounds.

Janet knows about the spread of sexually transmitted disease and has had treatment in the past. She associates AIDS with cancer, but understands the means of transmission of HIV and how to prevent the spread. She knows about AIDS from the television but had not spoken to anyone prior to the interview.

Janet was quite adamant that coloured men had brought the 'affection' (infection) to this country. 'AIDS kills, but there are tablets, needles and condoms to stop it.'

Teresa

Teresa is 29 years old. She is at present in the unit to which referrals are normally made from the courts, other hospitals or prisons. Teresa has been a resident for the last nine years, and has a history of drug use over the last 12 years. There have been several instances of her running away from the hospital to London and Wales.

Teresa told us that she had her first fix when she was in a squat in London and someone injected her. This led to a cycle of stealing, sleeping rough and squatting, which led inevitably to contact with the police. She has appeared in court for forging prescriptions, apparently as part of a criminal ring for the illegal procurement of drugs. A lot of her friends have died from drug use. She reports not having used drugs for some time.

Teresa's first sexual encounter was when she was 15. Later in her life, another woman had arranged for her to have sex with many partners in return for money and a roof over her head. Teresa also had sex for money to feed the children, who were not hers.

She first learned about AIDS from television and magazines several years ago, and she has extensive knowledge on the subject. This has led her to talk to a lot of people about it and further reading. She is extremely knowledgeable on the subject, making the ready link with hepatitis.

Her experiences with the police have all been bad, mainly due to her involvement in the drug scene. She would like to see drug users having ready access to free needles and syringes. Even though they know they should not share needles, drug users may do so if they are desperate for a fix 'because of the craving'.

Teresa has had regular sex partners and enduring relationships with other residents. Her last relationship ended when her friend was found dead in bed. During the interview, she told us that she was not allowed to attend the funeral because there were insufficient staff able to escort her! However, on investigating this with hospital managers, it was discovered that she did go to the funeral and that she chose not to go to the subsequent burial; there were no staff shortages. She still grieves for her friend and has visited his grave, which as yet does not have a headstone.

Sex is not important to her, but she is well aware of the means of contraception and doubts if many of the other residents have a clue about sex.

Alfred

The following case study concerns a member of staff. In line with the previous case studies, a pseudonym has been used.

Alfred has worked at the hospital for the last six years. While we were explaining the project, he volunteered that he was HIV antibody-positive. 'I wish someone had told me about HIV. I wouldn't be in the position I am now, taking AZT [zidovudine] every four bloody hours.' Alfred was happy to tell us of his experiences since he had found he was HIV-positive four years previously. He originally developed a rash on his shoulder which he showed to a doctor on the ward, who said she thought it was shingles. His GP, who was aware he was gay, said he had never seen such severe shingles and thought it might be Kaposi's sarcoma. The GP advised him to have 'the test'. If the result was negative, he would tell him over the phone. After ten days, Alfred was extremely concerned about his condition and wanted his results, but these eventually took five weeks to come through. When Alfred phoned and was asked to come into the surgery, he knew it was a positive result.

Alfred was offered but refused counselling support. He independently contacted the Terrence Higgins Trust and the Body Positive group but got no reply or support and, as a result, 'went into his shell'. After 18 months, he developed a chest infection and took up the offer of counselling. He was offered admission to his local hospital, but he declined because many of the staff would have known him. After an initial refusal, he was eventually admitted to a London hospital. He has now spent three periods as an in-patient, and is full of praise for the staff at the hospital. Alfred has been taking Zidovudine for the last year.

He was very lonely when he was an in-patient. He did not have many visitors, but felt he could not take the staff's time and attention when there were people around him in a worse condition. It was some time before he told his family, but they have been very supportive.

After his period in hospital with a chest infection, he informed his senior nurse manager of his health status. Alfred was moved to a rehabilitation ward (which housed patients who at some time or other had been violent) supposedly because of the risk of being bitten by patients on his former ward. Alfred began to have more time off to attend the hospital. On one occasion, when returning from out-patients in London, he met one of his residents who told Alfred that he knew that he had been in hospital in London. The resident had been told by a charge nurse who worked on the same ward that Alfred was very ill. This led to Alfred again being moved to another ward. Alfred now talks freely about his status. One or two members of staff were a little concerned at first, but, once they had learned about the illness, they were more supportive towards him. He feels that he should take a responsible approach and informs the staff with whom he works about his status, so that, in the event of an accident, they can take suitable precautions.

Alfred recently broke his ankle. When he presented himself to the Accident & Emergency Department of the local hospital, he told them that he was HIV antibody-positive. He reports that the casualty staff were 'brilliant' in the way they handled him, and that the sister asked if she could sit and chat to him because that was the only way she would find out about HIV infection.

His experience at the fracture clinic was very different. Apparently the doctor was only interested in his medication, which hospital he attended, whom he saw and what symptoms he had. The questions became so intrusive that Alfred refused to tell him any more. His ankle was eventually plastered. When he returned three weeks later to have the plaster removed, the doctor was brisk and offhand with him. He was reported as saying 'There is no need for physio. You will get enough chasing after the nutters at [the hospital]!'

Alfred is an ordinary person. HIV/AIDS has made him special. This attitude is brought about by the rareness of his disease and the response he is receiving from the staff at the hospital in London. Alfred is becoming involved in the local Body Positive support group.

His main concern is that the type of support he receives in London should be readily available locally. While we are only 18 minutes away from London by train, it is still expensive and an effort to get there, particularly if you are not feeling well. Alfred receives no financial supplement for travel because he is in full-time employment.

Depression is his worst problem. He has at times felt suicidal. He recognises that this was due in part to keeping the knowledge of his infection to himself. As a consequence, he is now happy to talk and tell people of his condition.

Alfred lives with a female friend in a deep platonic relationship. Alfred does not think that, in the past, he was particularly promiscuous. He claims that the press reports of gay men having many sexual partners during an evening or at an orgy are outside his experience: 'I was never so lucky!' His sex life has come to a complete standstill. Alfred wishes to die at home in familiar friendly surroundings. He says: 'Death does not bother me. It's how you die that does.'

Discussion

In the past, society has buried its head in the sand concerning the care of people with a mental handicap – out of sight, out of mind. 'Care in the community', a concept which has been with us for the last 20 years, is attempting to allow people with a mental handicap to 'come out' in several senses of the word.

HIV/AIDS has forced different communities to re-examine issues of and attitudes towards sexuality, and mental handicap institutions and communities are no exception. The issue of sex and people with a mental handicap is an extremely sensitive one. Views of the sexuality of people with a mental handicap can be divided into several camps, into which both staff and parents or guardians are divided. This is expressed by conflicting and polarised opinions such as: people with a mental handicap are children, innocents abroad; they have no sexual desire; they should not be allowed to reproduce for fear of diluting the genetic pool; they are unable to care for their offspring. Contraception and libido suppressant drugs have been proposed as an answer. There is also the argument that people with a mental handicap are sexually irresponsible and that we need to protect them from themselves for their own good and the good of society. There is also a fear that people with a mental hadicap are more likely to commit sexual offences, particularly against the young.

The segregation of the sexes that has occurred in many hospitals and institutions has led to many misconceptions concerning the practice and labelling of homosexuality. In a male-only world, how can a man express his sexuality other than by bonding in some way with another male, with varying degrees of homosexual practice and the sexual relief of masturbation? The only alternative may be abstinence.

The failure to mix the sexes gives individuals no chance to develop life skills and relationships with the opposite sex, based on choices and experiences. There is no opportunity to find out what 'normal' behaviour is.

Many adults have enjoyed reminiscing while reading about Sue Townsend's Adrian Mole and his adolescent development, but was it really so enjoyable when we were living through it? The frustrations, embarrassments, lack of confidence, difficulty in meeting members of the opposite sex, let alone talking to them in an intelligent, endearing way. Then there were problems of where to go for a kiss and cuddle – suddenly offering to babysit for your parents in order to get some privacy indoors with a girl or boy. This was also a time of experimentation and having multiple partners. Later on there were problems of where to go to be intimate – barns, cornfields, cars or bus shelters! With maturity and financial independence, most people overcome these problems, settling down in a long-term relationship or marriage.

This is not the case for people with a mental handicap. Our interviews have revealed that they remain in what only can be considered a permanent state of 'adolescenthood' in their sexual behaviour. There is nowhere to go for sex, no privacy – the only options being the cricket field, the bushes or the top of a hospital fire escape. Many residents reported, that they were not allowed to have sexual intercourse, or even to sit and cuddle on the wards or in the villas. However, it was allowed outside, whatever the weather, but not in front of the public. Social education is normally a skill that continually develops from early childhood; for people with a mental handicap, this has often been neglected.

One answer is to allow residents to express themselves sexually, to send them or allow them to go to hotels or guest houses together. As preparation for this, why not provide hotel-style facilities within the hospital grounds? This then raises questions of priority of use of limited facilities, abuse of the system by dominant residents or by staff and objections from the public, parents and guardians. It potentially leaves the authority open to charges of irresponsibility and brothel running. Surely a caring, non-judgemental system could be devised with both residents booking in, as would any normal couple at a hotel.

Many residents in conversations with us gave the impression that sex was only a means of gratification or to gain favour with other residents. All gave a history of sexual abuse of one sort or another, and they had a jaded and cynical view of sex. Their attitudes and approach to it had none of the sense of abandonment and enjoyment that a caring relationship can bring to the act of sexual intercourse. Development of more stable relationships could also lead to a reduction in the number of sexual partners.

Residents also associated sex with violence, either from their own experiences or the television. Due to their lack of social skills, they appear to be locked into a cycle in which they do not mix with the opposite sex and they are not taught about sexual relationships. A 'normalisation' programme for residents must provide the appropriate assistance in protecting themselves from HIV and AIDS. It must also accept that some people may be homosexual and will need support, assistance and direction to discover appropriate social venues.

Staff attitudes

The attitudes and opinions of staff who worked with some of the residents and patients were also sought, although not in a formal structured way. It was found that the more recently qualified staff had, in general, a more open and progressive approach to the residents' right to sex as part of their right to a normal life.

It is accepted that people with a mental handicap are easily influenced by their peers and carers. The carers have a basic responsibility to avoid sexual stereotyping. We gained the impression that this might be a problem from some of the residents' comments, such as 'Sex is dirty' and 'I had the baby taken away because I am not responsible to take care of it.' These statements seemed completely out of character when compared with the vocabulary they had been using during the interviews.

Almost all of the residents interviewed had a good knowledge of HIV/AIDS. They reported that this came mainly from the television. Very little seemed to come from the staff, although our involvement in this project may well have prompted staff to discuss some of the issues with residents. Within the hospital, there is a growing acknowledgement from some of the staff that every person with a mental handicap (resident, patient or client) has a right to express his/her sexuality. This, in turn, requires a planned sex education strategy with appropriate training for staff and residents. Hospitals should be preparing guidelines for staff on personal and sexual relationship education for residents.

The main message that the staff feel they need to get across to patients is contraception in general, leading on to specific HIV/AIDS education. It was generally agreed that patients with regular relationships should be supplied with a quantity of condoms to use as and when they choose.

Those responsible for developing sex education and AIDS education programmes must include the views and participation of parents and guardians. Because of the special needs of people with a mental handicap, the sex education programmes must be wide ranging and practical, including the questions of masturbation, petting and how to have intercourse, how to use a condom, sexually transmitted diseases, homosexuality, pregnancy and parenthood. It must also be acknowledged that normal relationships between both handicapped and non-handicapped people fail, break down and go through peaks and troughs which can cause turmoil and depression. Sex education and sensitivity to it are a responsibility for everyone and should be considered at staff selection, with ongoing in-service training and development programmes.

The health authority has a statement of philosophy with strategic and operational plans, policy documents and standing orders for procedures and staff guidance. Mental handicap units, institutions, homes and places of care must produce and observe similar policies and procedures.

Condoms

All people interviewed were well informed on the choices available for contraception and knew that condoms were available for purchase from the hospital shop. None, however, admitted to purchasing them. Residents who were sexually active and used condoms bought them at local chemists' shops. However, the women appeared to regard the fact that they were on the pill or had a coil fitted as sufficient protection against infection as well as pregnancy.

Most residents receive a Department of Social Security allowance of between £5–8 per week from which they are expected to purchase personal items and toiletries. There is not a lot left for condoms at 59p for a packet of three. Not many people would be prepared to spend almost 12 per cent of their salary on three condoms!

On further inquiry, it was found that condoms had only been on sale at the hospital shop for a few months and that only six packets had been sold – all to members of staff. While this initiative is to be applauded, there should be other outlets in the hospital and villas for residents to obtain condoms. The residents interviewed requested that condom vending machines be installed in the hospital social club. Even so, there is still the problem of the residents not having enough money to purchase condoms. The answer might be to install vending machines and have tokens freely available without charge from the bar, ward or hospital shop.

The fear that a black market in condoms might be created or the system abused by staff or residents hoarding or selling them would require some discreet monitoring. As long as the condoms are being used, it is better than unprotected sex and the risk of HIV/AIDS.

Further study

Our study by its nature gives only a snapshot view of the situation in certain mental handicap hospitals. We accept that the criteria for selection of residents for interview were biased, and would encourage a more in-depth study within our locality.

A three-year research project has been agreed with North West Thames Regional Health Authority, so that HIV/AIDS education programmes can be researched, devised and piloted, followed by the implementation of a programme for staff and residents' education. Care staff must be prepared and sensitive enough to provide assistance and guidance in creating individual sex education programmes.

Legal aspects

We have chosen in this paper not to enter into discussion concerning the minefield of legal issues about informed consent. (All the residents interviewed were considered by their care staff to be able to make an informed decision as to whether they took part in the study or not.) The legal framework will, however, have to be carefully considered in order to protect the residents, the staff and the authority.

Sex and the law

At present, there are seven statutes passed by Parliament relating to people with a mental handicap and sexuality (Table 16), as well as numerous reports, health circulars, DHSS memoranda, case law and committee recommendations, not forgetting any local Acts or bylaws that may be in force. Prosecutions under any of these Acts are likely to occur in a criminal court rather than a civil court. Some of the main issues that will concern authorities, staff and parents are: abortion, indecent assault, sexual intercourse and rape, homosexuality, masturbation, sexual relationships with staff, contraception advice to the under-16s, marriage and divorce, indecent exposure and sterilisation.

Table 16 **Statutes relating to sexuality and people with mental handicap**

Sexual Offences Act 1956
Mental Health Act 1959
Sexual Offences 1967
Mental Health (Amendments) Act 1982
Mental Health Act 1983
Sexual Offences Act 1985
Education (No. 2) Act 1986

The Sexual Offences Act 1956 states that it is illegal to have sexual intercourse with a 'mentally defective man or woman', and the Mental Health Act 1959 makes reference to staff having intercourse with female in-patients. While bearing the above legislation in mind, this, by the definitions used, leads to the labelling of people. The Family Planning Association Education Unit has produced an excellent guide, *Sex and the Law*, for anyone working in this field (Gunn and Rosser, 1987).

Nor have we investigated the physically disabled who also have a mental handicap – people who may need assistance from a third person in order to have intercourse with a partner.

Conclusion

The failure to recognise people's right to express themselves sexually, whatever their sexual orientation and preference, is to 'demote' them. This is even worse when it is coupled with the stigma attached to mental handicap.

We also recognise that, here, we have concentrated on high-risk behaviour between adults, but for many people with a mental handicap, as for non-handicapped people, relationships are not always sexual and intercourse does not necessarily occur.

People with mental handicap must be protected from abuse and exploitation. We have the right to choose. Equally, we have the responsibility to protect and ensure that the less fortunate in our society have the same choices.

Reference

Gunn, N. and Rosser, J. (1987) *Sex and the Law: A brief guide for staff working in the mental handicap field*. London, Family Planning Association.

Preparing the Way in Northern Ireland: HIV and AIDS and the Eastern Health and Social Services Board

Dr M. Paula J. Kilbane, Fiona O'Donnell and Dr Agnes McKnight

Northern Ireland has a population of some 1.5 million people in an area about 140 miles east to west and 90 miles north to south. It is predominantly rural apart from the eastern seaboard containing the city of Belfast with its population of 320,000. Traditional industries within the city include linen manufacture, ship building, cigarette manufacture and distilling. The city was in its industrial heyday in late Victorian times (Blaney, 1988), but many industries are now in decline.

Northern Ireland is divided into four health and social services boards: Northern, Western, Southern and Eastern (*see* Fig. 12). The Eastern Health and social services Board covers a population of 636,000, comprising about 41 per cent of the total in Northern Ireland, and is the most densely

Figure 12 Health and Social Services Board areas in Northern Ireland

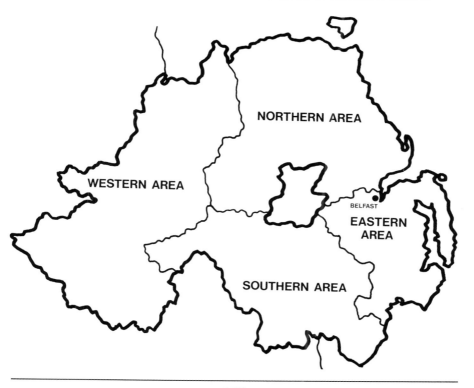

populated of the Board areas. The population is relatively young compared to that of the rest of the UK, with little projected increase by 1991. There is evidence of inner city deprivation and substantial unemployment. The overall level of unemployment is 20 per cent, but this may reach as high as 60 per cent in certain parts of Belfast. The area also has a greater proportion of semi-skilled, manual and unskilled people compared with Great Britain. There are few members from ethnic minorities living in the area.

Northern Ireland has a rather conservative culture. A very high proportion of the population are regular church goers. Surveys have shown that almost 40 per cent of the adult population abstain from alcohol (Harbison and Haire, 1982). The 1967 Abortion Act excludes Northern Ireland and the legislation in respect to homosexuality, which came into force in 1967 in the remainder of the UK, only became applicable there in 1982 as the result of a case brought to the European Commission on Human Rights. While little is known about sexual behaviour in Northern Ireland, some preliminary studies into student behaviour suggest that, among university students, sex and marriage are regarded as inseparable (Snedden and Kremer, 1988; Brown *et al.*, 1987). Just under 40 per cent reported ever having sexual intercourse, and few indicated having more than one partner. This compares with 78 per cent in a European university study (Clement *et al.*, 1984). Religiosity played a large part in explaining these findings, with frequent church attendance going hand in hand with sexual abstinence.

The civil disturbance over the past 20 years has meant that the influx of visitors and exchange of personnel between Northern Ireland and the remainder of the UK have been reduced. In addition, the high security profile has discouraged the smuggling of drugs, and the influence of paramilitary organisations in socially deprived areas is thought actively to discourage organised distribution and usage of hard drugs. In consequence, there is virtually no known heroin abuse in Northern Ireland. This is in direct contrast to the situation which obtains in the Irish Republic. There is a particularly serious problem in the Dublin area, where, it has been estimated, there are approximately 3,000 heroin users, many of them in the deprived inner city housing estates (Freedman, 1987).

There are good transportation and road networks in Northern Ireland, as well as two main airports. The ferry port alone handles about 1.5 million passengers a year. There is considerable business travel with over 250,000 outward journeys a year, 90 per cent of which are to England and Scotland. In the summer holiday season, about 150,000 people travel abroad. There is some anecdotal evidence that people from Northern Ireland may exhibit less conservative sexual behaviour while away from home either on business or holiday.

Organisational structures

There is no regional health authority in Northern Ireland. The regional function is provided by the Department of Health and Social Security, Northern Ireland (DHSS, NI), which is responsible for resource allocation, the production of strategic planning guidelines, and a wealth of information functions.

The Eastern Health and Social Services Board (EHSSB), with an annual budget of some £330 million, provides both health and social services for its population. For administrative purposes the geographical area is divided into 14 'units of management': some of these are acute units containing large teaching hospitals; some have both community and hospital functions; and others are of specialised nature, including, for example, psychiatric or mental handicap hospitals. The units of management serve populations varying from urban to rural and from 53,000 to 175,000 in number.

The EHSSB provides not only health services but a full range of social services including residential and childcare services, residential care for the elderly and handicapped, home-help services and meals on wheels. Each unit of management is responsible for the provision of services in its patch. The Board has a general manager, but the new general management structure has not yet been introduced down to unit level. The units are managed by 'unit of management groups'.

The EHSSB is a member of the European Group of Healthy Cities and is committed to collaborate actively with local authorities and statutory bodies. Health promotion and health education services are provided from within the Area Department of Community Medicine.

Local authorities are responsible for environmental health, and the Board itself liaises closely with two environmental health departments: Belfast City Council and the Eastern Group. The local authorities are also responsible for a number of other relevant services such as leisure and sport facilities and waste disposal. Housing is provided separately by the Northern Ireland Housing Executive.

Public education (apart from university education) is administered centrally by the Department of Education, Northern Ireland (DENI) and locally by five education and library boards (ELB), which are broadly equivalent to local education authorities in England and Wales. There are three main sectors of post-primary education:

- *Controlled:* managed primarily by ELBs; these are secular and largely Protestant.
- *Voluntary:* maintained schools managed primarily by boards of governors and, in the Eastern Board, by the Down and Connor Diocesan Board; these are largely Roman Catholic.
- *Voluntary grammar:* non-maintained and independent; these schools

can be Protestant or Roman Catholic.

The Central Services Agency is the equivalent of the Family Practitioner Committees in England. It provides services for the Boards on a regional basis, including payments to family doctors. At the present time, there are 383 practising family doctors in the Eastern Board, over half of whom work from 21 health centres and the remainder work from their own premises. Practice sizes are, on average, smaller than those in England and Wales. The GPs attached to health centres work closely with other members of the primary care team, some of whom are attached to a particular practice while others work on a geographical basis.

General practitioners' views are represented in many ways. There are GPs on the EHSSB and on area executive teams and within unit of management groups. Several are members of Northern Ireland's Council for Postgraduate Medical Education. The Royal College of General Practitioners has a Northern Ireland Faculty with 565 members. The British Medical Association has a structure here similar to that in the rest of the UK.

Prevalence of HIV infection and AIDS

Local clinicians and the Regional Virus Laboratory and Blood Transfusion Services report directly to the Communicable Disease Surveillance Centre (CDSC) at Colindale and to the DHSS, NI. The DHSS medical officer responsible for infectious diseases then alerts each health board with the numbers of new reports of AIDS or HIV antibody-positive test results.

The situation in Northern Ireland as of November 1988 was that there were 10 persons with AIDS and 49 who were HIV antibody-positive; 4 deaths from AIDS had occurred. This gave a prevalence for Northern Ireland as a whole of 6 per million for AIDS and 32 per million for known HIV infection. The numbers of persons being treated is higher than the reported case numbers due to the return home of some individuals diagnosed elsewhere. There is no evidence of others travelling to Northern Ireland to make use of services. Of those known to be seropositive, 21 were homosexual or bisexual men, 16 haemophiliac, 7 heterosexual (3 male, 4 female), 2 injecting drug users and 3 others. Precise local data about age are not available, but most infection occurs among young adults. It is estimated that the likely number of HIV-positive persons in Northern Ireland may range from 200 to 400, and future projections for people with AIDS for 1991 are between 45 and 75 (using UK estimates). In the Irish Republic, the number of known HIV antibody-positive persons is much greater (over 700), the majority (450) being injecting drug users.

There is a clear policy about testing and consent, but it is not possible to say how well this works except in certain closely controlled environments such as the genito-urinary medicine (GUM) department. Within the last year, the proportion of requests for HIV testing which came through this department constituted only about one-third of those performed by the Regional Virus Laboratory. The others were from primary care and hospital sources right across Northern Ireland.

AIDS: The initial impact

The local response to HIV was initiated on two fronts. First, there was the urgent need to provide testing services, both for blood transfusion and for those wishing to be tested at the GUM clinics and elsewhere. At the same time, the voluntary sector initiatives began – in the first instance, from Carafriend, one of the local gay organisations. Some preliminary discussion also took place between the area departments of community medicine and health education and the voluntary sector.

In the autumn of 1986, the Chief Administrative Medical Officer (CAMO) of the Eastern Health Board set up a series of expert advisory sub-committees to advise him on a comprehensive strategy for AIDS. The key individuals who were involved included those who were providing services for testing and for haemophiliacs, the GUM physicians and the Department of Community Medicine.

Structural responses

Following the Board's acceptance of this comprehensive AIDS strategy, a group known as the AIDS Steering Group was convened by one of the area specialists in community medicine in February 1987. The AIDS Steering Group was given the specific remit to secure the implementation of the Board's strategy. Within the Eastern Health Board, there has not been a proliferation of other AIDS groups or committees, perhaps because many of the local community and social services are also provided by the EHSSB.

The AIDS Steering Group is multi-disciplinary with membership from community medicine, nursing, dentistry, social services, planning, health education and clinical medicine (including a genito-urinary physician and a general practitioner) with co-option as required of finance and personnel representatives. Also included are two key personnel: the AIDS education co-ordinator specifically appointed by the Board, and the chairman of the voluntary AIDS Helpline. The role of the Group (summarised in Table 17) is, in essence, to ensure that the area strategic plan gets translated into action, and to report to the area executive team officers (and, through them, to the Board) on a quarterly basis.

The AIDS Steering Group functions very well and has not evolved significantly since its establishment. Key personnel have remained constant. Specific tasks have been tackled by small sub-groups rather than

Table 17 **Role of the AIDS Steering Group**

1 To secure the implementation of the Board's strategy on AIDS including:
  ● The development of a training strategy involving the establishment of AIDS education and awareness programmes for unit-based multi-disciplinary training groups within the Eastern Board.
  ● The development and dissemination of good models of practice for staff.
  ● Provision of appropriate out-patient and in-patient (short-term and long-term) accommodation.

2 To prioritise bids for resources for AIDS and approving allocations (within agreed AIDS resources) on behalf of the CAMO.

3 To develop the take initiatives in the wider Easter Board community including major agencies such as the education boards and trade unions.

4 To keep under review the Board's AIDS strategy and documentation.

5 To develop a positive relationship with the media.

changing the membership of the main group. The group is directly responsible for the planning of services including AIDS prevention. This has resulted in the emergence of new networks (with the voluntary sector) and the strengthening of old ones (e.g. Education and Library Boards and other sectors providing education).

The DHSS, NI committee on AIDS has a remit to oversee and co-ordinate activities throughout Northern Ireland. The CAMOs of all Boards are represented, together with a number of clinicians who are responsible for providing testing and treatment services, and there is also a health education representative. The Northern Ireland Committee on AIDS is also a source for receiving reports on developments from within DHSS London and on national policy.

There is now an active voluntary sector in the shape of the AIDS Helpline, centred on Belfast. This provides a confidential telephone advice and counselling service four nights a week, staffed by both men and women. The Helpline has close links with the statutory services and provides a befriending service for people with AIDS. Funding for the Helpline is mainly provided by DHSS, NI.

Policy responses

The EHSSB strategy is comprehensive, embracing policies on prevention, testing, acute care, continuing care, control of infection, confidentiality and employment. Some of these policies are very specific, some of them are broad. For instance, the control of infection policies are those formulated by the Advisory Committee on Dangerous Pathogens and St Mary's Hospital group, with only minimal adaptations for local use. The Board has an employment policy stating that no one shall be discriminated against in terms of employment on the basis of their HIV status. Other policies – for example, on confidentiality and community care – are as yet only very broadly defined. It is anticipated that further areas for policy development may arise within social services. While these are being comprehensively developed, many policies in the preventive field have been translated into action. The AIDS Steering Group is responsible for holding, updating and implementing these policies.

There is no designated programme director *per se*, although the responsibility for carrying out the task is vested with the Specialist in Community Medicine who chairs the Steering Group. The bulk of the co-ordination, particularly on the preventive front, is carried out by an AIDS education co-ordinator, a full-time post within the Area Health Education Department. This appointment has been critical to ensuring progress in this field. It was originally a two-year fixed-term contract from February 1987, but this has now been extended for a further two years and adapted to include the next phase of a youth programme.

The post holder has responsibility for developing, introducing and maintaining the preventive AIDS initiatives on behalf of the Board. This involves not only substantial administration but also the production of suitable materials and a major training and liaison role. It was envisaged that the nature of the tasks required might well evolve over time, hence the need for fixed-term contracts.

Caring for people with HIV and AIDS

The Royal Victoria Hospital in Belfast is the designated centre for HIV testing, out-patient care and in-patient treatment of people with AIDS or HIV-related disease.

People with HIV and AIDS are at present cared for in hospital in side rooms. It is intended to provide a minimal two-bed facility for those who require dedicated sanitary facilities. However, the philosophy (which has yet to be tested) is to care for people with AIDS in ordinary wards.

With the present small numbers, those who are acutely ill are managed in the designated centre. It is envisaged that, as soon as it becomes practicable and necessary, these patients should be cared for close to their own homes and community. The emphasis will be on out-patient and day care maintenance through the GUM clinic and/or haemophiliac clinics. whenever possible in any initiatives. A positive effort has been made to

The development of a community maintenance team, an outreach from the GUM clinic, is currently under discussion. While the aim is to make all staff aware of AIDS, it is unlikely that local numbers would justify training all staff to provide direct care at first. However, the evolving social services guidelines clearly identify the need for a small number of fostering families to be trained to care for HIV-positive babies when the need arises.

Terminal care arrangements are *ad hoc*. Representatives from the terminal care agencies have accepted an invitation to join the AIDS awareness training programme, and the local hospice has declared a willingness to care for people dying with AIDS. The voluntary sector is developing a buddying service, and the aim is to allow people to die in the community if this is their wish.

Funding and resources

In addition to those from existing budgets, separate recurring funds have been identified for the AIDS programme. The AIDS Steering Group processes the bids and allocates funding for various requests for AIDS-related posts and a variety of revenue and capital schemes. In addition, the chairman of the AIDS Steering Group prepares bids for AIDS money generally with each planning cycle. The voluntary sector is funded for the greater part from DHSS, NI but also receives money from other sources such as Co-operation North, occasional grants and donations; it is now also generating some money from seminars.

Non-financial resources, such as the staff and buildings of the GUM clinic, are shared, but there have been additional staff appointed specifically dedicated to providing services for HIV/AIDS. These include a clinical psychologist in the GUM clinic and additional social work, medical and nursing staff. During their working time, these staff also treat patients who are not HIV-positive.

The advent of HIV has highlighted the inadequacy of the existing services for genito-urinary medicine and has resulted in an increase in scientific and laboratory staff. Capital funds have been sought to extend the GUM clinic premises and also to develop a very small in-patient facility with single rooms for people with AIDS. In comparison with other places with comparable small caseloads, there has been less difficulty in obtaining resources from the EHSSB. This must be seen in the context of the Board providing services for the testing, diagnosis and treatment of the majority of cases arising in Northern Ireland, at least in the medium term.

Research

A number of research projects in AIDS-related areas are ongoing. There has been a survey of knowledge and attitudes among students attending at student health centres. This was part funded by the Board and has now been published (Brown *et al.*, 1987). The Department of Psychology at Queen's University Belfast also carried out a pilot study (which will now be extended) among students about their sexual behaviour. Within the Genitourinary Medicine Department, there has been a variety of studies including: a study of knowledge and attitudes of GUM clinic attenders; a study focusing on the sexual history, partners and practices of both gay and heterosexual attenders; a current study across all of Northern Ireland of the knowledge, attitudes and practices of HIV/AIDS-related issues among GPs; and a GUM-based voluntary seroprevalence study of GUM clinic attenders. In addition, various national studies related to opinions and behaviour have been established in Northern Ireland.

Prevention and health promotion

Prevention activities are not entirely separate from caring services because it is often appropriate to conduct both simultaneously (e.g. in the GUM clinic).

While it primarily provides a telephone counselling service, the AIDS Helpline also works closely with groups in the community. It is responsible for conducting education on safer sex among the gay community, and for organising seminars and workshops with outside groups. These are often within the voluntary sector but also involve employees of public sector organisations such as welfare officers from the civil service.

Pre-test counselling is available specifically in the GUM clinic as well as from all GPs. Due to the very small number of injecting drug users identified within the Board area, there is no injecting drug users programme. Therefore the issue of needle exchange, although discussed and positively received at the policy level, suffers from the practical difficulty of finding an obvious outlet.

Education links with schools, staff training, work with primary care, the media and so on will be referred to later. The responsibility for the establishment of these services lies very largely within the community medicine and health education departments. There is close liaison with local environmental health departments and, to date, that has been on practical issues such as guidelines for tattooists, acupuncturists, etc., or in collaborating in educational initiatives mounted by the local Institute of Environmental Health.

It is local policy to involve both the community and voluntary sectors encourage a pro-active and positive response by the local media, but this has met with only limited success. The appointment of a designated spokesperson goes some way towards dealing with media issues, but further work is needed in this field. The major thrusts, however, are in education for the Board staff of about 35,000 individuals and for school children.

AIDS awareness for health and social services staff

When work first began in 1986, we looked elsewhere to see what was being done. Whereas others were involved in crisis management, we found ourselves in the fortunate position of having time to plan and, with our known seroprevalence at a low level, the opportunity to influence the future. Partly because the Eastern Board is one of the largest public sector employers in Europe and also because we have the advantage of an integrated health and social services structure, it was clear that we needed to devise our own training model to suit the particular needs in Northern Ireland.

Our approach to training has been to base it on adult learning principles, using participatory methods. The training is learner-centred, recognising that individuals have valid knowledge and experience which in turn influences how they act and feel. By tapping into those resources we have developed a model which utilises individuals' skills and resources at local level.

The rationale behind our approach was based on the premise that, if we were to be effective in the long term, it was essential that responsibility and ownership for AIDS awareness lay with local management groups and was not seen as a central resource provided on a one-off basis. Also we had learned from experience that it is those who work locally who best know the needs and priorities of a particular area.

The model devised was based on the 'Training of Trainers' philosophy

Figure 13 **Organisation of AIDS Awareness Programme (EHSSB)**

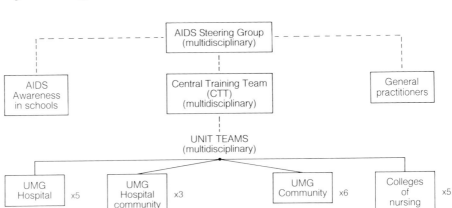

using a cascade approach. A multi-disciplinary Central Training Team (CTT) was selected and given a four-fold remit: to design and provide training for unit teams; to design appropriate training materials; to monitor progress; and to evaluate the effectiveness of the overall programme.

The training materials produced by the CTT for the unit teams took the form of a training manual. This contained medical facts about HIV and AIDS, methods and techniques for taking groups through AIDS awareness sessions, a section on values and attitudes, and further advice and support.

The unit teams were composed of staff from each unit of management. Their role, after they had been trained by the CTT, was to plan and provide training for all staff in their unit, thus reaching all 35,000 staff in the Eastern Board.

Because of their key role in health education and prevention, the colleges of nursing, the terminal care agencies and GPs were also included in the Board's overall AIDS Awareness Programme. For practical purposes, an additional model has been designed for GPs.

The Board's aims in providing AIDS awareness for all staff were: to raise their personal awareness about the risk of contracting HIV infection; to reduce to a minimum any occupational risk; and, by ensuring that staff were fully informed, to maintain high professional standards of care given to people with HIV infection or AIDS. In the overall context of the Board's strategy, which includes educating the public, it was also recognised that staff have a potential role in the education of the community. It was acknowledged that the additional skills acquired by the unit teams would be of lasting benefit to the unit of management within which they worked.

The primary concern was that those in the unit teams should have the confidence and skills needed to undertake the training of others. It was unlikely that many would have had formal training in how to work with groups, and only some would have had experience of planning education programmes. The multi-disciplinary nature of the teams was also a new way of working for many.

The first stage in preparing for the task was to assess the needs of the unit teams and the needs and priorities of their units of management. From the information gained, it was possible for the CTT to assess the kind of training package required. Consequently, training was offered in three stages:

(1) *Working with groups.* This was a two-day course which gave participants an understanding of group process, and confidence in running their own sessions. The course explored and developed an appreciation of the skills required to work with adult groups.

(2) *AIDS awareness.* This was a three-day course designed to help the team work together and allowed them to explore their own values and attitudes. It provided them with up-to-date information on the virus and its transmission and, finally, an opportunity to formulate plans for

implementing AIDS awareness locally.

(3) *Presentation skills.* This two-day course took participants through the practical skills of presentation. This was an optional course for those who felt they needed additional support in this area.

Overall, 70 trainers were trained over an initial period of six months. Since then, an additional 50 people have been trained to supplement some of the teams. Once teams started taking AIDS awareness sessions, they were assigned a trainer from the CTT for ongoing support and advice. This also acted as a direct source of feedback for the CTT and, ultimately, the Board. Teams communicate with each other and share their successes and difficulties through regular networking meetings.

An education programme on this scale had never been attempted before by the Board and presented many challenges. In the planning stages, and indeed throughout, we were concerned about many things. Would all units of management participate? Was the issue being taken seriously enough? Would the unit teams be able to do this task along with their other commitments? Was it possible to do this in a multi-disciplinary fashion? And, of course, would it make any difference?

With each unit of management being independently managed, the degree of commitment has varied. However, all 14 units have a team currently providing training, all the colleges of nursing have taken steps to train their colleagues and to introduce AIDS awareness into the curriculum, and the terminal care agencies have staff trained in anticipation of their key role in community care. We attribute our success so far to a number of factors. Before any models were designed or any training began, the strategy was in place and there were clear objectives. We consulted with management and the unions in the early stages, which gave them the opportunity to influence the proceedings. The trainers from the units were given a comprehensive training package, including help with preparation for planning and prioritising, along with built-in ongoing support networks. Part of the strategy identified a need for a post with the specific remit to co-ordinate the activities of the Board on AIDS/HIV. Finally, the commitment of certain individuals and the loyalty of the members of the unit teams have played a crucial role in the success to date.

With the relevant skills and experience, we had the ingredients of a credible programme. However, the difficulty of staff in the units finding time for planning and training amid their other commitments has been an ongoing problem. It has been met, in some instances, by management releasing staff from some of their normal duties, but staff still find that some of the administrative work of training is done in their own time. In recognition of this, the AIDS Steering Group released one-off sums of money to each unit to assist with the additional administration.

The multi-disciplinary nature of the teams has worked extremely well. Members of the teams have reported a great deal of satisfaction from working in a multi-disciplinary setting, and have described how the experience and contact with other disciplines is having a direct benefit on other aspects of their work. Some difficulties did arise where others' perceptions of the team did not meet with traditional expectations – e.g. non-medical staff taking a session on AIDS. This has been dealt with on a local basis, usually offset by management intervention. However, with hindsight it is clear that a wider use of circulars and more explicit memos to introduce each team and their role would have been useful to enhance their credibility.

One thing we did not adequately anticipate was the effect of success and its implications for the workload on the CTT. As each team started work, and word passed from each unit of management, more people joined the unit teams. This, in turn, meant providing extra training, and, since the CTT were also providing the ongoing support, this was a considerable extra load.

In raising awareness about the transmission of a sexually transmitted disease, the training addresses sexual behaviour and its role in prevention. Although this was accepted by the CTT as a logical inclusion in training, this was not always accepted by those who received the training – something that may seem obvious to those who have been working on an issue for some time may not always be obvious to the uninitiated. Although incidents of this kind have been rare, the few that have arisen have caused setbacks in morale. As a result of this feedback from participants, our training package now places a greater emphasis on context setting and the rationale behind the training.

As a low-prevalence area with many other high-priority health issues, there was a chance that this issue would not be given serious attention. As a result, our AIDS awareness programme for staff has been likened to a 'low birth-weight baby' – 'low birth-weight' because the odds were against it surviving birth. However, the programme has been given a safe delivery and is now in its incubator being nursed to greater independence. An independent evaluation of the programme has been commissioned, but until the survey produces some concrete evidence, we have only the subjective feedback from the recipients of the training. This seems to indicate that the programme will survive to adulthood.

AIDS education in schools

In January 1987, discussions were initiated between the EHSSB and representatives from the education sector on the promotion of AIDS awareness for young people. From these discussions came a multi-disciplinary writing group to produce AIDS and HIV teaching materials for use with 14–19-year-olds in Northern Ireland schools. The composition of the writing group includes representatives from community medicine, health education, school health, teaching, a moral philosopher, the

Northern Ireland Council for Educational Development (NICED) and the voluntary sector AIDS Helpline.

A literature and resource review of current educational material was carried out to assess its suitability for Northern Ireland schools and colleges. Those that were available were considered only partly suitable for a society which is generally conservative, in which sexuality is a sensitive issue, where there is relatively little officially recorded drug use, and where there is adverse reaction to those who are gay. Northern Ireland is also a low-prevalence area for HIV infection, which could have made it more difficult to get the issue recognised as a priority over so many other health concerns. The joint writing group was given a remit to produce suitable piloted materials and have a product available to schools for the academic year 1987–8.

A teaching pack – *AIDS Education for Schools* (1988) – was produced in March 1988. It contained a teacher's handbook, a set of reinforced pupil material for photocopying, materials for card games, and transparency masters for overhead projection. Since much of the package dealt with attitudes and feelings, an active learning approach was employed throughout. Guidance was given to teachers on the application of this approach, with methods and materials appropriate for each activity.

The questions we asked ourselves before writing the pack were centred on our concerns about the possible barriers to the successful implementation of the materials in the schools. In a society whose culture is dominated by religious teaching, it was not assumed that there would be immediate acceptance of the introduction of this issue into the school curriculum, and we were also unsure about the possible reactions of parents and leading public figures. Ownership of the pack was another major concern – would something which was initiated by a health board be acceptable to the education sector?

To take account of these concerns, we organised a two-pronged approach. The AIDS Steering Group and the joint writing group worked in parallel, and while the latter got on with writing, the former conducted a consultation process which was to set the climate for acceptance once the materials were produced. Communication between the two groups was maintained through the person of the AIDS/HIV co-ordinator. The Northern Ireland Council for Educational Development (NICED) is a body with a specific remit to develop educational material and in-service training in schools. NICED played an important role in the development, training and dissemination of the pack throughout Northern Ireland, and has agreed to take responsibility for publishing the pack. The timetable for the project is summarised in Table 18.

The initial consultations were held with the general manager and chairman of the EHSSB, the chief officers from the education and library boards (ELBs), representatives from the Down and Connor Diocesan Board and the Governing Bodies Association, in order to reach agreement from the outset about the importance of AIDS education in the curriculum. At a later stage, the consultation meetings were extended to include education advisers and school principals. The process of updating continued throughout the year that it took to produce the pack. Because of their role in supporting teachers in schools, the school health team were also given briefings and updates on the progress of the pack. It was anticipated that these people would be a crucial support to teachers once they were using the materials in schools, and particularly with parents' meetings.

The pack is designed to be used where work on sex education has already been undertaken. It may also be included with an integrated health education programme, as part of a general studies course, or integrated into subject teaching where, for example, the medical content could be covered in biology and the moral and ethical issues discussed in religious or social studies.

The aims of the pack were: to provide accurate factual information about AIDS and HIV infection; to encourage the pupils to explore their attitudes to disease and personal relationships; to promote responsible behaviour based on self-respect and respect for others; and to identify sources of help and advice in the community outside the school.

There are three units in the pack, each outlining activities for two class sessions. In the first unit, the pupils are helped to understand the defence systems of the body, to obtain knowledge about infections and transmission, and to identify HIV/AIDS as a sexually transmitted disease. The second unit aims to identify existing knowledge, to consider the myths and misinformation and to present accurate information about HIV and AIDS. The third unit uses small group work and discussion to explore attitudes, and moral and social issues. This unit requires sensitive leadership, and it is crucial that it is taken in an atmosphere of trust and mutual understanding. At the beginning, attention is drawn to the necessity that teaching within this unit is consistent with the ethos of the school.

Before using the pack, teachers were offered a two-day briefing programme on the application of the approach and the materials appropriate for each activity. Two places were offered to each school initially. A complimentary copy of the pack was given to teachers who attended the training, while each principal was already in receipt of a copy. Attendance at the in-service training has been unprecedented. In the Eastern Board's area, 76 per cent of post-primary schools have had one or more teachers trained, the special schools have had 45 per cent and the colleges of further education have had 62 per cent.

We have been successful in getting the pack into the schools, and the ownership of the pack is firmly established in the education sector. We are awaiting evaluation of the feedback from teachers who have used the pack in the schools. Only then will we be able to assess the extent to which the

Table 18 **Implementation of the schools pack on AIDS awareness, Eastern Health and Social Services Board, NI**

Month	Steering group activities	Writing group activities
January 87	Review of literature and resources.	Multi-disciplinary writing group formed.
February 87	Brief produced for writing group.	Writing began. Group divided into 3 working groups.
March 87	Met the chief education officers from both ELBs. Representatives from Down and Connor Diocesan Board and Governing Bodies Association. This meeting hosted by Area Executive Team of EHSSB.	Sub-groups met regularly to feedback on progress.
May 87	Met with education advisers from both ELBs. Seminars for school principals held to inform them of plans, outline pack and to accept practical or moral objections at this point.	Draft materials near completion.
June 87		Teachers from pilot schools trained in use of the draft materials. Six schools took part in pilot.
August 87	Members of Steering Group and writing group met with Director of NICED. Agreed that they should be responsible for dissemination of package throughout NI. NICED agreed to co-ordinate publishing of pack.	Materials being rewritten in light of pilot.

Month	Steering group activities	Writing group activities
September 87	Seminars organised for school health staff to brief on pack and on their possible roles.	
October 87	Update meeting for those who attended first meeting in March. CEOs, Down and Connor Diocesan Board and Governing Bodies Association.	Rewritten materials produced in draft form.
November 87	Update meeting for those who attended the meeting in May. School principals from both ELBs. Chaired by CEO. Previewed draft materials.	
December 87	NICED begins process to involve other education and health boards in NI.	
January 88	Pack sent for printing. NICED negotiate cover leave for 2-day training.	
February 88	Schools sent advance information about pack.	
March 88		Writing groups and education advisers plan training for teachers.
April 88	Cover leave granted for 2-day training for teachers.	Training of teachers in the BELB and SEELB.
May 88		School health staff given printed pack and informed of schools in area who had taken advantage of the training and therefore likely to be looking to them as resource.

pack is being used.

The extent to which we consulted with key personnel and the fact that this process has been ongoing are the two major factors leading to the successful implementation of the pack. Also, as with our model for training staff, it is the commitment and motivation of particular individuals which have stood out when considering success. The multi-disciplinary nature of the writing group and the combination of relevant skills and personalities produced a very co-operative and productive team.

On a more pragmatic note, the reason why teachers accepted the pack so readily has been attributed to the fact that they felt comfortable with the materials after the training. In addition, the style of the pack meant that everything was included without the need to look elsewhere for background knowledge and supplementary materials.

As a direct result of the training, teachers from special schools voluntarily formed a working group to adapt the pack for use with children with special needs. This version of the pack is now also available to teachers.

The success of the schools pack has given impetus for further work to be done on sex education in schools. It is thought that this has only been made possible by the positive climate that has been created by use of the AIDS pack.

AIDS awareness in general practice

The greatest problem with initiating new ideas or change within general practice is the fact that GPs themselves are independent contractors and often work in relative isolation. There has been, in the past, a noticeable lack of funding for preventive services within the primary care setting, although it is hoped that this is going to change as suggested in the Government's recent White Paper *Promoting Better Health*.

The AIDS Steering Group is committed to establishing AIDS awareness in general practice and, to this end, has a GP as one of its members. A sub-group of GPs has been looking at ways in which various aspects of AIDS awareness could be promoted within the setting of general practice, with particular reference to attitudes to confidentiality and procedures (handling specimens, needles, waste, etc.).

Two projects have been initiated with GPs. First, there has been a survey of all GPs in Northern Ireland to establish their attitudes to, and knowledge about, HIV infection. The ultimate aim is to design a programme appropriate to their demonstrated needs. The response has been good, and preliminary analysis suggests that GPs feel that they are lacking in skills, particularly in relation to the counselling issues around HIV and AIDS.

The second project aims, in part, to respond to the first. Approval has been given for a two-session appointment of a general practice facilitator whose role will be to develop, in conjunction with the AIDS Steering Group, an AIDS awareness package for primary care. A pilot meeting in a large health centre attended by all members of the primary care teams of four practices has taken place. Educational films were shown and small group discussions took place. This was moderately successful, but it was felt that a series of meetings of smaller groups (comprising a maximum of 20 individuals) might be more beneficial. Certainly it was considered important to have the members of the team working together in any discussion. The details of the facilitator post are still under discussion. Possible options are for a GP to take on the role or even to split the post and create a small multi-disciplinary team.

Obviously the time required for such an individual training programme will be lengthy. We strongly feel that any approach to GPs other than a personal one is unlikely to succeed. It is interesting to note that other health education and health promotion activities being organised by the Eastern Board – e.g. cervical and breast screening, childhood immunisation programmes – are using the individual approach and sending 'action teams' out to the GPs in their workplaces to promote these activities.

Efforts by education-promoting organisations, such as the Northern Ireland Faculty of the Royal College of General Practitioners, the Ulster Medical Society and the Northern Ireland Council for Postgraduate Medical Education, have already been made to promote AIDS awareness. Several seminars for GPs have been held and more will be strongly encouraged.

Courses for general practice receptionists are currently being held by the Northern Ireland Training Council for Health and social services with help from the BMA and RCGP. These are to be continued and widely promoted.

Conclusion

Where activities have been successful, this was due to taking advantage of successful joint initiatives that had occurred before and convincing key people at the top of the particular organisation (e.g. general managers) of the importance and urgency of the issues. Enlisting people with already proven credibility was important; we had the advantage of having certain people within the EHSSB who have a very finely developed strategic sense and who thus gave very appropriate advice. Having such a varied management structure in the schools, we were very conscious of the necessity to produce flexible materials in consultation with all three main sectors (*see* p. 159). It was emphasised during negotiations and training that the pack should be used in a way which was consistent with the ethos of each school. Very few problems about differing philosophies and territorial issues have occurred to date, but these may very well surface later.

As far as problems are concerned, we have not managed to cope with all the prejudices and ignorance. This has been most difficult when it is found in key individuals who may not even be aware of their own prejudices.

Homophobia is very deep rooted in Northern Ireland, people do not 'come out', and a lot of time needs to be spent on emphasising risk *behaviour* as opposed to risk *groups*. There were also, initially, problems in trying to get local units to take ownership of AIDS training without significant additional resources, although the legislation in respect of AIDS has been a great help in promoting AIDS awareness in the workplace. We have given a little funding to individual units, but the resources required to do that properly are enormous and we will never be able to meet them.

Some media responses have been very good – others, from predictable sources, less so. While the prevalence remains low in a population of this size, cases of AIDS will always give rise to adverse and unwanted attention. However, the low prevalence has given us the opportunity to take time and develop pro-active responses which we believe will influence the course of the epidemic in the future.

References

AIDS Education for Schools: A Northern Ireland package on AIDS awareness for schools. (1988) Eastern Health and social services Board, and Northern Ireland Council for Educational Development (NICED).

Blaney, R. (1988) *Belfast, 100 years of public health.* Belfast City Council and Eastern Health and social services Board.

Brown, J. S., Irwin, W. G., Steele, K. and Harland, R. W. (1987). Students' awareness of and attitudes to AIDS. *Journal of the Royal College of General Practitioners*, 37, 457–8.

Clement, U. *et al.* (1984) Changes in sex differences in sexual behaviour: a replication of a study on West German students (1966–81). *Archives of Sexual Behaviour*, 13, 99–120.

Freedman, D. (1987). *AIDS: The problem in Ireland.* Town House, Dublin.

Harbison, J. and Haire, T. (1982) *Drinking Practices in Northern Ireland.* Policy Planning and Research Unit, Department of Finance and Personnel, Northern Ireland.

Sneddon, I. and Kremer, J. (1988) *Sexual Behaviour and Attitudes in Northern Ireland – a pilot study of a student sample.* Department of Psychology, Queen's University Belfast.

Health Promotion Responses to AIDS in Wales: The Welsh AIDS campaign

Virginia Blakey, Richard Parish and Debbi Reid

Health promotion is concerned with the creation of a social and economic environment which will foster healthy lifestyles. It involves the population as a whole in their everyday lives, and is directed towards action which will affect the determinants of causes of health and ill health. The support of health professionals in this endeavour is clearly important. However, it also requires close co-operation among a wide range of sectors and agencies, beyond those with specific responsibility for the delivery of health services.

Health promotion draws on a diversity of complementary approaches to achieve its goals; these may encompass mass media campaigns, legislation, fiscal measures, organisational change and community development, as well as more formal educational activities. A key component of health promotion is health education, which is concerned with increasing individual knowledge about health and illness, raising awareness about social and environmental factors that influence health, and helping people to acquire skills which will enable them to make choices and take action to achieve a healthy lifestyle.

HIV infection and AIDS pose a particular challenge in the context of health promotion. Because HIV infection is transmitted through sexual contact, health promotion programmes in this area have to deal with issues of sexuality and specific sexual behaviour. This is a very sensitive task, as most people regard sex as an extremely private area of life where intervention from outside agencies is inappropriate. The fact that AIDS was at first seen as an illness which affected mainly gay men has added a further dimension of difficulty, as has the link with injecting drug users. The public need to be made aware that the issue is one of risk behaviour, not risk groups, but the skills needed to lead discussions focused on sexual behaviour are in short supply. Delicate decisions have to be made about the content of leaflets and mass media messages, and some degree of controversy and public outcry is inevitable, given the plurality of values within our society. To a far greater extent than with some other diseases, individuals can protect themselves from HIV infection by making choices about the way they behave – but, first, they have to be convinced that this is a problem which has relevance for them.

Here we review the history of the Welsh AIDS Campaign, which has now become the AIDS Programme of the Health Promotion Authority for Wales (HPAW). Attention will be focused on the development and direction of the programme, its relationship with other statutory and voluntary agencies, and its response to the particular social and cultural factors prevailing in Wales.

Setting the scene

Wales is a constituent country of the United Kingdom, with a population of 2.8 million. It has the same legal system as England, but a separate government department, the Welsh Office, is responsible, *inter alia*, for health, education and local government within the Principality. In respect of the administration of these services, Wales is independent of England, although it frequently follows the policy decisions taken by the lead Departments of State in Whitehall.

Within Wales, there are 8 county councils, 37 district and borough councils, 9 district health authorities (7 of which are coterminous with the counties) and 8 Family Practitioner Committees. In addition to the statutory services, it is usual for each of the UK national voluntary agencies and professional associations to have a separate Welsh organisation and identity.

Although Wales does not have a regional health authority, some regional functions are performed by the Welsh Office, and some by district health authorities. Within the Welsh Office, there are a number of divisions which have an important part to play in strategic policy formulation. In addition to the nine district health authorities, Wales has two special health authorities: the Welsh Health Common Services Authority (WHSCA), which is responsible for a number of support services across the Principality; and the Health Promotion Authority for Wales, which was constituted in April 1987, at the time of the Health Education Council's reconstitution as a special health authority itself.

Economic and social characteristics

Gross domestic product (GDP) per head of population is the second lowest among the regions of the UK, being higher only than Northern Ireland. The last decade has seen a major decline in the traditional industries of South Wales – namely, coal and steel. The average unemployment rate in Wales since 1986 was the third highest regional rate, after Northern Ireland and the North of England. Much of Wales is rural in nature, and agriculture, forestry and fishing remain important industries and sources of employment.

Most parts of Wales exhibit a strong community identity and many aspects of Welsh life are more traditional than those in England. More marriages are solemnised by religious ceremony than in any of the English regions, although the illegitimacy rate is approximately the same, varying considerably, however, between the more rural areas (where it is low) and the major conurbations.

Although use of the Welsh language has declined during this century, there were still over half a million Welsh speakers in Wales (18 per cent of the population) at the 1981 census. The greatest concentrations of Welsh speakers are found in North and West Wales.

Response to the problem

Early concern about the AIDS epidemic in Wales was sparked off late in 1982 when a case was diagnosed in a young haemophiliac. Initial guidelines for AIDS surveillance were issued by the Welsh Office in May 1983, and these were followed in 1984 and 1985 by further circulars giving general information to doctors and setting out infection control guidelines for the community care of people with HIV or AIDS.

At this time, responsibility for advising the Welsh Office on health education issues lay with the Health Education Advisory Committee for Wales, HEAC(W), whose membership linked into a number of health networks and whose secretariat was located in the Health Policy Division of the Welsh Office. In September 1985, HEAC(W) set up a special sub-group to provide advice on the health education response to AIDS in Wales. The specific remit of the sub-group was:

- to advise HEAC(W), the Welsh Office and other interested parties on the health education response to AIDS in Wales.
- to respond to and initiate constructive media interest in the health education aspects of AIDS.
- to establish links with statutory and voluntary groups and other interested bodies to provide rapid feedback on needs and perceptions of the problem.
- to consider health education needs in Wales and, in particular, in conjunction with the Welsh Language Panel, advise on the need for Welsh language material.

Members of the group drawn from HEAC(W) included the chief administrative dental officer for South Glamorgan and East Dyfed health authorities, who was chair of HEAC(W) and the AIDS sub-group; the chief administrative medical officer for West Glamorgan Health Authority; the chief executive of the Welsh National Board for Nursing, Midwifery and Health Visiting; and the deputy head of a comprehensive school in Gwent. In addition, a number of people were co-opted to the sub-group, including: the district health education officer for South Glamorgan and a health education officer from West Glamorgan (who had both been carrying out AIDS education work in isolation in their respective counties); a specialist in community medicine from South Glamorgan; a GP from East Dyfed; and the director of the Sociological Research Unit at University College Cardiff, who was already carrying out research on sexual behaviour and AIDS, and had links with the gay community. The sub-group also had access to the expertise of an epidemiologist from the Public Health Laboratory Service.

Initial awareness of the impact and implications of HIV infection and AIDS was no greater in Wales than elsewhere in the UK, but the fact that the HEAC(W) machinery was available meant that the response within the Principality to the educational challenge posed by the epidemic was fairly swift. This was particularly so in view of the low reported incidence of HIV and AIDS within Wales at this time: by the end of 1985, five people with AIDS and three cases of HIV antibody positivity had been reported from Wales to the Communicable Disease Surveillance Centre at Colindale.

As an initial task, the sub-group considered the essential elements which would be required to underpin the governmental initiative on AIDS information. They therefore reviewed communication approaches through statutory and voluntary bodies and the media; health promotion materials available within the UK and abroad, both of a general nature and those aimed at specific target groups and voluntary agencies; and evaluation issues which would need to be addressed by any AIDS education campaign. As a result of this review, the sub-group identified a number of priority areas for action in Wales to complement the UK campaign. These were:

- a conference on counselling and confidentiality.
- a research programme to evaluate the campaign.
- telephone information and advice lines.
- publicity materials in English and Welsh.
- a media workshop.
- workshops for teachers and other professionals.

In February 1986, the sub-group made these recommendations to HEAC(W) in an interim report, which was then referred to the Welsh Office. The minister responsible for health at the Welsh Office accepted the group's broad conclusions in June 1986. By this stage, however, the UK government's own information campaign and the national helpline initiative were underway, and the minister requested that the sub-group provide more details on their proposals for a health education campaign and an associated helpline facility within Wales, noting that it was important that any initiatives in Wales should complement the UK-wide campaign and incorporate lessons from other parts of the world.

While these aspects of the sub-group's report were considered in more detail, other activities recommended by the group got underway. A training seminar for AIDS counsellors was held in September 1986, a pack for journalists was put together and a media workshop was planned for October 1986. At the same time, other proposals were being put to the Welsh Office. A member of the sub-group had attended the Second International Conference on AIDS in Paris in June 1986. Through contacts made there, he and the deputy chief medical officer of the Welsh Office made a fact-finding visit to the United States in September 1986 to review the experience of AIDS education in New York and New Jersey. The report of this visit included a proposal for the establishment of an independent AIDS foundation for Wales, which would mobilise community networks, set up 'taskforces' aimed at professional and voluntary groups, instigate a broad range of mass media activities and establish a Welsh data base for AIDS.

The approaches advocated in the two reports were in broad agreement; the question facing the Welsh Office was how the AIDS education initiative in Wales might best be taken forward. Having given consideration to the prevailing climate of opinion, it was felt that a separate campaign might be the most appropriate vehicle, as it would have an independent identity which would enable it to be more effective in spreading the necessary educational messages.

As a result, the Welsh AIDS Campaign was launched on 1 October 1986, to coincide with the media workshop. The members of the HEAC(W) sub-group, with their range of different skills and networks, were to continue to direct the campaign, with a full-time co-ordinator to implement the programme. The campaign had the following remit:

- to provide up-to-date information to the public, professionals, media and other interested groups concerning AIDS.
- to seek through health education to modify personal behaviour to lessen the risk of contracting or spreading HIV.
- to seek to alleviate unnecessary anxiety concerning AIDS through the provision of timely and accurate information.
- to provide advice and guidance concerning AIDS on request to individuals and groups.
- to provide training to volunteers, health educators and other profession-als in providing advice concerning AIDS prevention.
- to promote consistency in the 'message' on AIDS presented to the public and interested groups by the media, professionals and others working in the field.

The launch of the campaign received extensive press coverage and aroused a great deal of interest within Wales, to the extent that expectations were generated which it was almost impossible for the campaign to meet. In order to get the work of the campaign underway, premises had to be found, administrative and secretarial staff appointed, and equipment and resource materials purchased. In the initial months of the campaign's existence, these tasks took up a great deal of the co-ordinator's time. The appointment of administrative support in January 1987 alleviated some of this pressure, but still left more work than could be covered by available staff resources. The campaign was also deluged with requests for talks on HIV and AIDS from a variety of groups. This externally determined workload meant that the campaign activities took on a reactive rather than a pro-active character – a difficulty reported by similar agencies in other countries during the early stages of public response to the epidemic. The process of mobilisation and networking was inevitably slowed down, and this led to some difficulties with voluntary and professional groups which hindered the work of the campaign.

The setting-up of the campaign also coincided with the preparatory stages of the first UK government mass media initiative. On 12 January 1987, the campaign initiated a telephone advice line to provide backup information to the government leaflet drop throughout the UK. A rota was organised by the district health education officer for South Glamorgan, a member of the HEAC(W) sub-group, and, with the help of suitably trained volunteers, the campaign dealt with 3,000 telephone calls over a three-week period. A third of these calls came from outside Wales.

A particular difficulty arose in finding premises for the campaign. Suitable accommodation was located in a multiple-occupancy building and a leasing agreement had been finalised when the other tenants discovered who their new neighbours were to be. As this was at a time of mass hysteria about AIDS in the press, there was considerable opposition and public outcry. In the end, alternative accommodation in a hospital site was obtained, but the incident created difficulties for the campaign and was a further setback.

In spite of these problems, some very good work was achieved by the campaign during its first few months. The co-ordinator put a lot of energy and enthusiasm into talks to many different groups and into responding to media requests for information, ensuring that the issue of AIDS was kept in the public eye. A survey of knowledge and attitudes about HIV and AIDS among the people of Wales was commissioned from an independent market research agency; the initial research, carried out in December 1986/ January 1987, provided an invaluable baseline of knowledge against which to compare the results of later similar surveys (*see box*). A leaflet designed to inform young people about HIV transmission and prevention was produced, and was well received in other parts of the UK and overseas as well as within Wales.

Using research to direct programme activities

From its inception, the Welsh AIDS Campaign has used regular tracking surveys to monitor public knowledge and attitudes about HIV infection and AIDS, and has drawn on the findings to guide programme activities. Since March 1987, surveys based on home interviews with a representative sample of 1,000 adults in Wales have been conducted every six months. These surveys have addressed a range of issues relating to HIV and AIDS, including knowledge of transmission, perceptions of 'risk groups' and 'risk situations', and attitudes towards HIV infection and people with AIDS.

Results from the surveys have shown that correct knowledge of the main modes of transmission is high (96–97 per cent), but have also pointed up a number of misconceptions about potential infection among a minority of respondents – e.g. that HIV can be spread through kissing or sharing utensils. Findings have highlighted the difference between apparent knowledge about HIV infection and genuine understanding of the nature of the disease, raising important issues for public education campaigns.

The survey results have also indicated some interesting changes in attitudes towards the disease and those affected by it. Prejudice against people with HIV infection has declined, particularly among women. However, 1 in 5 respondents still have serious reservations about people with HIV infection living in the community normally or about working alongside someone with HIV infection. As a result of these findings, the promotion of sound workplace policies in this area is becoming an important part of the Health Promotion Authority's AIDS programme. Staff are also giving even greater stress to the accuracy, sensitivity and consistency of language and images used in health promotion work relating to HIV and AIDS.

A further trend revealed by the surveys has been a decline in fatalism about HIV infection: the majority of respondents believe that most people should be concerned about the disease and doing something to prevent its spread. In the September 1988 survey round, only 12 per cent of respondents agreed that 'AIDS is only a problem for homosexuals and drug abusers', and only 10 per cent agreed that 'Heterosexual men and women don't need to worry about AIDS.' However, the data have also shown that, in spite of identifying sexually active heterosexuals as being potentially at risk, very few respondents apply that risk to themselves. These findings have made it clear that having information about HIV infection is not enough to reduce risk behaviour; people also need to see the issue as one which applies to them. During 1989, the Health Promotion Authority will be giving even greater support to community-based educational initiatives and to the use of experiential learning methods, in an attempt to bridge this gap between theoretical awareness of the facts about HIV infection and actual changes in individual behaviour.

Six months after its launch, the Welsh AIDS Campaign was affected by changes in the national structures relating to health education. The government's decision to reconstitute the Health Education Council as a new Health Education Authority led the Welsh Office to consider the future of HEAC(W). Plans for a Health Promotion Authority for Wales, which had been previously discussed as a possible future development, were given more urgent consideration, and the decision was taken to set up the new HPAW during 1987. On 1 April 1987, the Welsh AIDS Campaign became the responsibility of the new Authority, whose chair (Dr Simon Smail) had been chair of the HEAC(W) sub-group since June 1986.

The setting-up of the new HPAW inevitably entailed a slowing in the momentum of the campaign, as it took time for the organisational structure of the HPAW to be finalised and for new managerial and financial arrangements to be agreed and put into effect. Nevertheless, by the end of its first year, the Welsh AIDS Campaign had achieved the following goals:

- publication of two market research studies on knowledge of and attitudes on AIDS throughout Wales.
- a series of seminars and study days for statutory and voluntary workers throughout Wales:

March 1987: 1-day conference for nurses
April 1987: 2-day residential conference for DHEOs
May 1987: 1-day conference for drugs fieldworkers
July 1987: 1-day conference for drugs fieldworkers
2-day introduction to basic counselling for helpline volunteers
follow-up day for drugs fieldworkers
September 1987: follow-up day for DHEOs
November 1987: 1-day conference on 'AIDS in the Workplace' for trade union members
1-day course on 'Social and Emotional Needs of People who are HIV-Positive' for representatives from statutory and voluntary groups.

- the development and up-dating of an information pack to accompany each of the training sessions.
- development and dissemination of the leaflet *AIDS: What it means for young people.*
- regular attendance at meetings of district health authority AIDS co-ordinating teams throughout Wales and at meetings of DHEOs.
- presentations about the work of the campaign at various international conferences in Europe and the US.

An education and training officer was appointed to the campaign in September, enabling closer links to be forged with voluntary groups and with health education officers with responsibility for HIV/AIDS.

The current situation: some key issues

With the integration of the Welsh AIDS Campaign into the Health Promotion Authority for Wales (HPAW), some significant changes have occurred in the way that the AIDS programme is implemented.

One advantage of the new structure is that staff from the four specialist divisions of the HPAW – operations, research and information, communication and community affairs, resource and development – are available to implement different aspects of the authority's operational plan, according to their particular areas of expertise. Thus, the tasks of developing a database on HIV/AIDS, carrying out research and monitoring the programme's effectiveness have been undertaken by the research and information division; advice on dealing with the media is supplied by the communications and community affairs division; and work with local education authorities and other local authorities is being carried out in consultation with the health promotion advisers within the operations division who have special responsibilities for these networks. The demands which this organisational strategy poses in terms of communication and co-operation between staff of the HPAW is considerable, but this advantage is hopefully outweighed by the gains in flexibility and specialist knowledge.

A further area requiring frequent consultation and sensitivity about boundaries between areas of responsibility is the relationship between HPAW and the district health authorities within Wales. The need to co-ordinate activities has been a concern since the establishment of the Welsh AIDS Campaign, and the Welsh Office has sought to provide a framework to achieve this through the circulars which have been issued on HIV and AIDS. In particular, key circulars asking district health authorities to develop co-ordinated plans for services (May 1987) and giving guidance on the way forward in developing services (August 1988) have made reference to the role of the Welsh AIDS Campaign or HPAW's AIDS programme, and have sought to encourage consultation.

HPAW's role is to work on an all-Wales basis in a way that complements and enhances the activities being carried out at a district level, for example through conducting relevant research and providing information and training support to professionals, and by developing, supporting and publicising pilot projects which may provide a model for district activities. Successful fulfilment of this role requires consultation with district health authority AIDS co-ordinating teams (ACTs) and with district health education or health promotion units. Staff from the AIDS programme aim to visit ACTs at least once a year, with more frequent informal consultation on specific issues. Meetings with district health education officers are held several times a year to ensure that operational plans and programme activities are complementary and mutually supportive. Frequent information exchange meetings also take place with health education officers with responsibility for AIDS work.

HPAW also has a distinct role to play in relation to macro-level organisations within Wales – that is, all-Wales bodies of varying descriptions, for whom issues of professional training or workplace policies relating to HIV and AIDS may be particularly significant. A current example of this role is HPAW's collaboration with a working group of senior staff from local authority social services departments within Wales who are developing a training strategy on HIV and AIDS for social services staff. In terms of HPAW involvement, two issues are of importance here. First, the timing must be right; both the professional group concerned and their employing authorities must have reached some degree of internal consensus on the need for HIV/AIDS training. Second, staff from HPAW's AIDS programme need to be aware, and to show that they are aware, that the group or organisation with which they are working has a professional perspective on the issue which will, to some extent, shape the content and method of any training. HPAW's role is to provide appropriate input within that professional context, not to impose an externally determined training package.

A further specific role allocated to the programme is that of liaison and collaboration with the Health Education Authority in England. In addition to regular quarterly meetings of AIDS workers from the four national bodies with responsibility for health education and promotion, consultations on issues such as publications, research and targeted programme activities take place frequently. A particularly important area for liaison is the mass media public education campaign on HIV and AIDS. While the HEA has responsibility for this campaign on a UK-wide basis, HPAW has the task of advising on the appropriateness of the material from the point of view of Welsh society and culture. HPAW is also concerned with the adaptation and translation into Welsh of HEA materials on HIV and AIDS, as ensuring availability of appropriate materials in Welsh is an important part of HPAW's remit. Following discussions with teachers and health educators in Welsh-speaking areas, HPAW has commissioned a Welsh version of the HEA schools pack *Teaching about AIDS* to meet the needs of young people in these communities.

Co-ordination with the voluntary sector is also of key importance. Prior to the integration of the Welsh AIDS Campaign into HPAW, the campaign's offices were located next to those of the Cardiff AIDS Helpline. This enabled the campaign's education and training officer, who was later appointed as the HPAW's health promotion adviser on AIDS, to build up a close working relationship with helpline workers, including the Welsh representative on the Network of Voluntary Organisations on AIDS and HIV (NOVOAH) and the National AIDS Trust. The health promotion adviser on AIDS regularly attends meetings of the Wales Voluntary AIDS Forum. She is now also a volunteer with Cardiff AIDS Helpline, and this has provided the AIDS programme with excellent feedback on the concerns of the voluntary sector, particularly with regard to training and support issues. HPAW is also represented on the Welsh Advisory Committee of the National AIDS Trust, which provides further useful insights into the needs and concerns of the voluntary sector.

Staff of HPAW's AIDS programme are committed to strengthening links between the statutory and voluntary sectors, and to encouraging joint working whenever possible. One way of promoting this is by combined training events, such as the workshop on 'Sexuality Awareness and AIDS' held in June 1988, which was attended both by health education officers and by helpline workers. Another is to emphasise the potential of voluntary organisations as sources of expertise. An example of this approach is the involvement of the Wales Family Planning Association in an all-Wales workshop for local education authorities on use of the *Teaching about AIDS* schools pack.

Factors affecting success

As this account has shown, development of the work of the Welsh AIDS Campaign and HPAW's AIDS programme has not been without problems and difficulties. The launch of the initial campaign raised expectations among both statutory and voluntary sector agencies which could not be met with the available staff and resources. Relationships with a number of statutory and voluntary groups within Wales also suffered initially because of the campaigns's inability to meet all the needs of these agencies.

The integration of the campaign into the new Health Promotion Authority for Wales, and the changes in personnel and organisation of work which this involved, also affected the morale of campaign staff and slowed momentum, particularly during the period when staff were located on different sites. Within the HPAW, the AIDS programme was faced with the task of clarifying and renegotiating its role *vis-à-vis* district health education units and other statutory and voluntary agencies. This meant that time had to be spent in rebuilding networks before programme activities could again get underway.

In spite of these difficulties, the AIDS programme has some solid achievements to show from the past two-and-a-half years. A number of factors can be identified as having contributed to this success. First, the fact that the Welsh AIDS Campaign developed through the established machinery of the Health Education Advisory Committee for Wales ensured a well-co-ordinated start to the programme. The campaign also enjoyed initial ready-made access to statutory networks within Wales through the members of the HEAC(W) sub-group. Support from the Welsh Office for the role of the campaign and then for HPAW's AIDS programme, through the framework of official circulars, was also very important in facilitating the programme's links with the statutory sector, particularly the district health authorities.

From its inception, the campaign enjoyed good relations with the media. The co-ordinator quickly established himself as a spokesman on AIDS-related issues, ensuring a high profile for the campaign's activities. The Chair of the Health Promotion Authority, who also chaired HPAW's AIDS Programme Advisory Group up to the end of 1988, is also frequently asked by the press to comment on new developments.

A final advantage has been the programme's close relations with the voluntary sector. Through networks involving members of the HEAC(W) sub-group, the Welsh AIDS Campaign benefited from good initial contacts and collaboration with the gay community in South Wales. Contacts with helplines and other voluntary sector organisations have been strengthened and extended by the health promotion adviser on AIDS, through her professional and voluntary activities.

All these factors have worked to the advantage of the programme, by enabling it to network effectively throughout Wales, a crucial task for an organisation operating at a regional level. As a result, the programme is now in a position to build on past achievements and to pursue vigorous and innovative programmes in the three areas which have been highlighted for the 1989/90 operational plan: public education, professional support, and promotion of workplace policies relating to HIV and AIDS.

The authors would like to express their thanks to Mr Bob Goosey (District Health Education Officer, South Glamorgan Health Authority) and Dr Simon Smail (Chair, Health Promotion Authority for Wales) for assistance received in the preparation of this case study.

Reference

Nutbeam, D., Smail, S. A., Catford, J. C. and Griffiths, C. Public knowledge and attitudes to AIDS, *Public Health* (in press).

The Challenge of AIDS – towards a model for a public health response

Dr Maryan Pye

Here we look at some definitions and models of health promotion and public health. A model of public health which encompasses health promotion is used as the basis for reviewing and commenting on the responses described in the previous sections. A final summary proposes ways in which districts can assess their current position with a view to planning for the future.

In January 1988, the ministers of health of over 130 countries met together in London to consider the worldwide epidemic of HIV infection and AIDS. One of the recommendations of the conference is summarised in what has become known as the 'London Declaration' about the prevention of AIDS:

> *In the absence at present of a vaccine or cure for AIDS, the single most important component of national AIDS programmes is information and communication because HIV transmission can be prevented through informed and responsible behaviour.*
> (World Summit of Ministers of Health on Programmes for AIDS Prevention, London, January 1988; Article 4)

The stated UK government public health strategy to combat the spread of HIV infection here contains the following elements:
- services for people with AIDS and HIV.
- specific measures to control the spread of HIV infection, including the screening of blood, tissue and organ donations.
- education aimed at the general public as well as people at particular risk.

This strategy has been translated into action not only by the development of central policy and the allocation of earmarked funding, but also through a wide range of initiatives at national and local level. This book concentrates on the responses at local level, particularly in the field of health promotion and in the development of new models of care and partnerships between agencies.

Definitions and models

In an analysis of these local responses, it may be helpful to consider HIV/AIDS as a public health problem requiring, to a large extent, a health promotion approach. Public health has been defined (in the Acheson Report) as 'the science and art of preventing disease, prolonging life and promoting health through organised efforts of society' (DHSS, 1988). 'Health promotion' is itself a term used in a variety of different ways. The Health Education Authority has defined AIDS health promotion as 'the culture-specific process which seeks to influence positively the relevant health practices of individuals and groups so as to minimise HIV transmission without harmful social impact.' This definition is all-embracing and yet lacks specific content since the nature of the 'process' is not defined.

Green and Raeburn (1988) have discussed the limitations of the traditional behavioural/lifestyle approach to health promotion when it is divorced from a social or 'systems' model which considers the social, economic, political, institutional, cultural, legislative, industrial and physical environments in which all behaviour takes place. They advocate an integrated approach in which the concepts of 'community' and 'enabling' are crucial elements in linking individual behaviour and environment. Such conceptual models are helpful in recognising the need to involve and empower people in the definition and improvement of their own health, but provide little by way of a framework for reviewing the process.

Tannahill (1985a) proposed a model of health promotion comprising three overlapping spheres of activity – health education, prevention and health protection (Fig. 14). The first two of these activities are generally well understood. 'Health protection' parallels many aspects of the systems model outlined above, in that it covers legal and fiscal controls, other

Figure 14 **A model of health promotion**

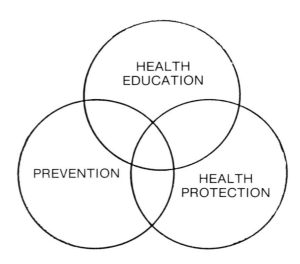

regulations, policies and codes of practice which in turn create an environment which may hinder or facilitate the enhancement of positive health and/or the prevention of ill health. A detailed description of this model entails an examination of the activities represented by the areas of overlap, but this will not be pursued here.

It has subsequently been suggested (Tannahill, 1988) that this model is also applicable to the concept of public health, although it might be argued that it does not adequately demonstrate the activities relating to the provision of appropriate care which are essential to the public health response. However, controlling the epidemic of HIV and AIDS is quintessentially a public health problem, and the model (with some modification) provides a practical basis for analysing the range of responses to this challenge.

Incorporating models of care

The sphere of activity described as 'prevention' has traditionally, and somewhat artificially, been subdivided into primary, secondary and tertiary prevention. There is broad agreement on the concept of primary prevention as avoidance of the onset of disease, and secondary prevention as early detection and treatment at a stage when serious consequences can be avoided. Tertiary prevention has been defined both as the alleviation of discomfort and disability in chronic disease which cannot be cured, and as the management of established disease to avoid or limit the development of disability or handicap.

Since treatment is aimed at preventing certain consequences of the disease state, it has been argued that this may be sufficient justification for considering all treatment within the concept of 'tertiary prevention' (Tannahill, 1985b). While this has the advantage of semantic tidiness, it demeans the extent to which specific expertise has developed in the care of people with HIV/AIDS. There have already been clinical and pharmacological advances in the management of HIV-related disease and innovations in the ways in which care is provided, both in hospital and in the community. For the purposes of this analysis, 'care' is considered as a separate field of activity, encircling and overlapping the other aspects of public health.

Other dimensions of public health

There are two further dimensions to be considered (Fig. 15). We have looked generally at the responses of organisations, sometimes working independently, but often working in concert. Public health responses are usually mounted in the context of social organisational frameworks, the dynamics of which may or may not be enabling.

The other dimension for consideration is time, both in the historical sense of observing change retrospectively over time and also representing the current position in relation to the progress of the epidemic. The epidemic curve in the UK has until very recently shown little change from that originally observed in the United States. At any point in 'historical' time, people may be addressing problems posed by different stages in the progress of the epidemic.

Figure 15 **A public health model for the response to HIV/AIDS**

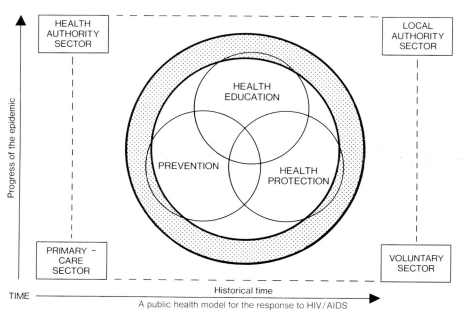

A public health model for the response to HIV/AIDS

Time and the epidemic curve

The various responses and initiatives described in this book have to be seen in the context of their timing. The case studies have provided a brief introduction to each district and an indication of its position on the epidemic curve. This, in turn, has influenced what local initiatives have been either possible, appropriate or both. In areas such as Wales and Northern Ireland where the prevalence of HIV/AIDS is currently thought to be very low, there has been a particular emphasis on education and preparation for what now is seen as inevitable. As we have seen, it has required considerable effort to persuade the relevant parts of the organisational framework that there is merit in a pro-active approach to prevention by means of education and training, as well as to give priority to the planning of care and treatment services for people with HIV-related disease. The natural history of HIV infection is such that preventive action today will not alleviate the burden of disease for tomorrow, although, if effective, it should reduce the incidence of AIDS several years hence.

In some districts, a high prevalence of HIV infection has already led to a high incidence of AIDS. The pattern of infection in these districts is similar to that experienced in the United States where early cases were largely confined to the homosexual population. In the UK, this pattern is seen in urban areas such as London and Brighton with large gay populations. As in the United States, awareness of the means of transmission of the virus has led to marked changes in the behaviour of gay men in this country, which will reduce the risk of further spread. However, we cannot afford to become complacent about the effects of changed behaviour: there is worrying evidence from Brighton that the previously observed reduction in sexually transmitted disease has not been maintained. For districts with a heavy clinical workload of HIV-related disease, the prospect of health education for primary prevention may be in danger of being considered something of a luxury and accorded lower priority than the initial 'fire-fighting' responses.

Other centres show different patterns of infection due to local factors. For example, Oxford and Bradford are the sites of regional units for the care of people with haemophilia. From the national data, it appears that these districts are the sources of a disproportionately high concentration of reports of HIV infection acquired from blood products.

From Lothian, we see yet another aspect of the epidemic, in which the known prevalence of HIV infection is high, but the incidence of AIDS is as yet low. This represents an earlier point on the epidemic curve, and we can predict that there will be a rapid increase in the number of people with AIDS in Edinburgh in the next two or three years. In the east of Scotland, the proportion of drug users who are antibody-positive is much higher than any recognised in the rest of the UK, and this suggests that the progression of the epidemic in Scotland may take a different course.

Taken overall, a few committed individuals in the lower-prevalence districts have had to stimulate interest and recognition of the need for action, but there has been the opportunity to examine models of care based on experience elsewhere, before agreeing major resource commitments. At the same time, these 'second wave' areas are able to share with the high-prevalence districts their new expertise in training and education which has been arrived at through innovative but rational and well-thought-out routes.

Time and history

The other aspect of time to be considered is the broad historical perspective. The contributions from Paddington and Bradford give contrasting historical accounts of the development of local initiatives in the light of the prevailing pressures which constrained or promoted that response. In Paddington, a high-prevalence district, the problem of AIDS was primarily a clinical problem to be addressed, at least initially, by the provision of appropriate hospital care, but, over time, the power base for decision-making and resource allocation has shifted. (The experience in Bloomsbury has been similar and has been summarised elsewhere [Ferlie and Pettigrew, 1988].) In Bradford, without the pressures of a clinically led service, but with a tradition of collaborative working with the local authority, the opportunity was taken to develop a response to HIV infection which mirrored the outbreak control process for other epidemics of infectious disease. It is as yet too soon to consider whether this process will alter with the change in political leadership of the local authority.

Organisational frameworks

The responses described in this book are not individual or personal, but involve the reactions and interactions of organisations or groups of people. For the most part, the organisational response is from the National Health Service, and there have been responses by way of funding and guidance from central government. Regional health authorities are involved in the allocation of resources to districts and, more recently, are acknowledging their role to co-ordinate action between districts with the development of regional strategies and health promotion programmes.

The case study reports are mostly seen from a district health authority viewpoint, and its interactions with the local authority sector, the voluntary sector and primary care. Although general practice is part of the health service, it is not within the span of control of the district health authority.

There are a number of common responses which have been initiated in most districts, but often we see that similar initiatives have been developed by different agencies – for example, the lead agency in community care may be the voluntary sector, the primary care team, or health and/or social services.

Organisational responses to public health issues traditionally involve the health and local authorities, but, in the case of HIV and AIDS, the role of the voluntary sector is particularly prominent. In London voluntary groups such as the Terrence Higgins Trust were, at a very early stage, the mainstay of health education, care and support which they continue now through sponsorship by, or as the agents of, the statutory sector. The London Lighthouse arose as a voluntary initiative, although it is dependent on grants from statutory bodies for its survival. It is an example of the voluntary sector leading the way in determining the style, level and quality of care which can and should be provided for those with life-threatening disease. The lessons to be learned from the initiatives of organisations such as London Lighthouse are relevant to many different groups in society and not solely the province of those with HIV-related disease.

Almost all the case studies make reference to the role of the voluntary sector helplines, and there is no reason to believe these districts are not typical of the UK as a whole. In most instances, it has been groups from within the gay community who have organised telephone helplines to provide advice and counselling and who have then brought pressure on the statutory services to respond. In some districts, there have also been responses from voluntary agencies working in the drugs field. As a result, some imaginative and creative partnerships have been developed with the statutory sector. In Brighton, for instance, the Sussex AIDS Centre and Helpline is no longer seen as an exclusively gay organisation; it has expanded and employs full-time workers in order to undertake training on behalf of the local authority and to provide a centre for day care.

In theory, mechanisms exist for health and local authorities to collaborate on issues such as community care as well as on aspects of environmental health and infectious disease control. There are statutory structures for the joint planning and funding of initiatives which involve the health services with their corresponding environmental health, social services and education departments. The voluntary sector is formally represented in this process. In practice, however, the effectiveness of this joint planning process is extremely variable, often dependent on the degree of coterminosity of the geographical boundaries of the contributing organisations, and perhaps reflecting the personal energy, enthusiasm, expertise or charisma of the individuals involved.

The complementary way these groups can work together effectively is demonstrated by the jointly planned and funded schemes for care in the community and housing for people with mental handicap or the elderly.

An example of a successful joint planning mechanism is in North West Hertfordshire which has recently expanded to include joint planning teams for health promotion and HIV/AIDS. In Brighton, the AIDS Liaison Group is an important link in co-ordinating prevention and care services and is structurally part of the joint planning mechanism. Another instance of collaboration is the AIDS Forum in Bradford, established under the auspices of the Metropolitan District Council, reporting to the Public Health Subcommittee but with membership and involvement of all interested parties. By way of contrast, in Oxford, the District AIDS Taskforce was an essentially health service-based group with little in the way of formal structural links. However, good co-operation was maintained with the local authority through the innovative joint appointment of an AIDS liaison officer and also the unusual local arrangement by which the health education service is jointly managed by the health authority and the local education department.

In central London, where there is a lack of coterminosity between the statutory organisations involved and a less well-defined sense of community, the joint planning process does not appear to work so well. The two London case studies reveal the difficulties of attempting to co-ordinate care outside the hospital for people with HIV-related disease. The report from

Paddington relates the history of repeated attempts to convene the appropriate joint planning forum. However, there is no doubt that the teams working at the individual client level in these two districts are finding ways around the problems.

Some organisational difficulties arise because the different sectors do not always understand the ways in which the others work. Voluntary agencies are usually innovative and enthusiastic and find it hard to understand the resourcing, time-scale and policy issues which constrain larger bureaucratic organisations in the statutory sector. Similarly those working at the individual client level, whatever their base, may consider a population-based approach unduly constraining and perhaps contrary to the client's interest.

There is always the possibility of conflict between planning authorities and the people, i.e. practitioners, who directly provide care to individual clients and patients. Practitioners may have legitimate priorities and preferences in this work which are different from those of the individuals and groups responsible for creating strategic plans. Implementing these plans may prove to be difficult if they require changes in the behaviour of practitioners. Conversely, practitioners who experience at first hand the needs of people with HIV-related disease may become very frustrated by the inability of the health and local authorities to provide facilities in time to help an individual patient.

These difficulties are brought into sharp focus by the independent contractor status of GPs. Because of this status, there is no line management which can direct them to respond to the challenge of the HIV epidemic in a particular way. As a consequence, marked variations between GPs are apparent whatever performance indicator is selected. The reports in this book reflect the highly individual nature of primary care services and the difficulty of negotiating a range of services with a number of independent contractors, none of whom can ever be said to represent the interests of the others. This is a continuing problem for general practitioner representatives on planning teams and committees. A feeling of frustration comes through from individual GPs who are committed to working with people with AIDS; they mostly have to bear the brunt of criticism of their colleagues who may be less enthusiastic about working in this field, perhaps because they are less well informed. Nevertheless, the independence of general practice has enabled the pioneer GPs to be effective advocates on behalf of their patients in identifying deficiencies in the range of services available.

There are probably as many different organisational responses as there are localities. What seems to be a common factor for success is the establishment of a group or groups which represent all interests and which have an identified route to executive action. A pre-existing foundation for collaborative working is also advantageous, but this can be achieved in a variety of ways. In densely populated areas such as London, this approach may be less successful due to the lack of coterminosity of the agencies involved and the very strong hospital lead for service provision. There is also a potential disadvantage when the AIDS initiative is steered mainly by a group which serves as a focus for policy development but may have little direct power or access to resources.

Having considered the framework and time scale by which any response may be constrained, it is appropriate now to consider the broad spheres of activity which comprise the public health response:

- *Health protection*, in creating the environment for change.
- *Prevention*, as the measures taken to prevent further transmission of the virus.
- *Health education*, to encourage and sustain appropriate changes in behaviour.
- *Provision of appropriate care.*

In the original description of his model, Tannahill emphasised the positive health-promoting nature of some areas of activity and made clear distinctions between the activities represented by the different areas of overlap. However, the purpose of this review is not to provide a detailed analysis according to the subtleties of the model, but simply to refer to the content of the case reports within the broad framework outlined above.

Health protection

This can be summarised as the area of activity which influences the climate in which responses to the epidemic of HIV/AIDS may be facilitated or hindered. In other words, it represents the politics of the situation.

The climate of public opinion is fluid and changes over time. It is influenced by the media, politics, education and prejudice. It provides a backcloth to local responses and can be influenced locally.

In the UK, a significant role has been taken by central government. An early response was to mount a mass media campaign which, despite its critics, served to make the public aware of the existence of AIDS and demonstrated the government's commitment to respond. Even before this, there were a number of funding initiatives and directives to the NHS, but again it has been argued that, when the money came, it was too little and too late.

The earliest funding initiatives of all came as research grants and were never intended to provide routine clinical services. Government funding followed in a piecemeal fashion, as earmarked sums to be allocated against various bids. There was no overall strategy or promise of long-term funding which might provide the basis for the rational planning of service expansion. Thus the method of funding served to distort priorities at the local level and caused particular conflict when new monies were made available in districts which were struggling with overspending problems. With the development of regional and local strategies and the promise of more long-term funding, the situation is becoming less fraught.

In addition to ensuring adequate funds, the ideal climate for change is one in which there is a clear statement of objectives, and an agreed strategy as the basis for preparing and implementing local operational plans. Reading through the case studies, it is possible to get the impression that the logic of this process has been inversely proportional to the clinical load. In high-prevalence districts, policy formulation began with infection-control guidelines to staff, and only much later has agreement been reached on a district strategy for responding to AIDS. For example, in Brighton and Paddington a range of practical guidelines and infection-control polices preceded the development of district strategies in 1988. An advantage to the lower-prevalence districts has been having time to agree a local strategy in advance, as was done in Northern Ireland and North West Hertfordshire in early 1987.

The reactions of the medical profession also influence both public opinion and organisational responses. In the early days, it was the medical staff of the London teaching hospitals who played a major role in publicising the potential severity of the epidemic and the need for a co-ordinated response. A less fortunate event, not specifically referred to in the case studies, was the debate surrounding the issues of consent and testing for HIV antibodies. The British Medical Association and the General Medical Council have subsequently produced clear ethical guidelines to the profession about informed consent, confidentiality and the duty to care. However, studies suggest that there is still an element of distrust which has to be overcome before GPs can provide the best care for their patients.

Pre-existing clinical policies also influence the possibility of change. During the 1970s and early 1980s, consultant psychiatrists responsible for drug dependency units moved away from policies of maintenance prescribing towards a goal of abstinence. There is an inherent contradiction between this philosophy and that of needle exchange schemes providing safer drug use. Successful schemes acknowledge this potential conflict and may actively negotiate ways for those ascribing to different philosophies to work together. Alternatively, such schemes are defined quite separately from the statutory medical drug user services and have strong community links.

Another aspect of health protection is the legislative structure, and we have had some examples where this might prove to be a hindrance. Prisons are designated as public places and, since homosexual acts are illegal in public, there has been an official reluctance to acknowledge the need for the provision of condoms, although the prison service has accepted the need for health education for staff and prisoners. The case study from North West Hertfordshire made passing reference to the legislation surrounding sex and mental handicap. The practical difficulties of introducing appropriate sex education and AIDS education into a large residential hospital stem as much from the culture of the institution as from fear of legal action. The response will have to appeal to the strategy of 'normalisation' and work through changing staff attitudes before individual residents can look forward to a more normal sex life. In the districts where needle exchanges have been established, there has been an explicit approach to gain co-operation from the local police.

What comes across from all the case studies is that there are a number of different ways of achieving the same ends. There is no 'right' way, but the best way is to understand the prevailing climate of opinion and to identify and work through key people. If the bases of power and knowledge can be involved, they can be used to create the demand, whether it be for service development or an educational programme for schools.

Health education

Health education can be described as activity which aims to influence the knowledge, beliefs, attitudes and behaviour of individuals or groups. The case studies in this book describe a number of initiatives in local health education. These can be loosely classified as health education in schools, for groups with special needs, for staff in an occupational setting, and some particular examples of work with general practitioners.

This is by no means a comprehensive classification of health educational approaches to HIV/AIDS. Almost all local health education/promotion units will be involved in a wide range of educational responses to AIDS. The aims of HIV/AIDS education are to provide information in such a way that people feel able to maintain or adopt behaviour which will reduce the risk of transmission of the virus. They also need to understand the nature of the infection and how they can best help those who are infected. For many people, this means that they will have to examine their own attitudes to sexuality, to risk-taking, and their own prejudices.

The detailed educational methods used and the evaluation of their effectiveness are not considered here. We are more concerned to examine ways in which such a sensitive educational exercise can be mounted to reach such a variety of audiences in such a relatively short time period.

The Health Education Authority (HEA) has a national responsibility for HIV/AIDS education. Although it is responsible for mass media campaigns aimed at the general public, many of its other activities are geared towards identified target audiences, but the response at local levels is limited to providing support. For example, HEA has recently launched a teacher's pack of materials for HIV/AIDS education in schools and supporting training, but this has come too late to support the initiatives described in our case studies.

It is clear from the case studies that it is the approach to working in schools which is almost as important as the curriculum content. One such example is the experience from Northern Ireland. The particular religious and cultural sensitivities and the varied management structure for education were recognised. Considerable energy was directed towards achieving consensus about including AIDS in the curriculum as well as developing the materials themselves, and the inclusion of a moral philosopher lent credibility to the writing group. Those not directly involved and who might have been concerned about divorcing the issue from a social or moral context felt reassured that someone was competently representing their concerns.

The method of dissemination described in Belfast represents a common thread through all schools initiatives. In the early days, health educators were inundated by requests for talks from schools. The inappropriateness of and lack of resources for this response have led to what would seem to be a universal approach. This recognises that AIDS education is not a separate subject, and that it has a place in the curriculum alongside other aspects of personal, social and health education. As such, it is best undertaken by the regular staff of the school. The role of health educators is therefore to work with teachers to ensure that they have the knowledge, skills and confidence to teach in this difficult area. What has emerged from 'training the teachers' is that this subject has to be handled sensitively, using active learning methods. Many teachers felt initially uncomfortable with these methods, but, with the help and support they received in this process for AIDS education, many now feel better prepared and more willing to tackle other sensitive subjects such as sex education.

It is essential that any local initiative takes into account the particular sensitivities of the local population. In Bradford, the Community Health Initiative has been established to work with the Asian ethnic minority groups. One problem is the absence of educational materials for those whose first language is not English, but this is greatly complicated by the fact that there are cultural differences which make it quite inappropriate, even offensive, merely to translate the educational programme into a different language.

The project in Bradford is an example of community development methods in health education. If we are to achieve our aims of influencing attitudes and beliefs about HIV/AIDS, we will need to work more closely with communities to help them identify the problems from their own perspectives and to work with them in developing responses which fit with their priorities and values. Community development methods are an area for potential growth in developing holistic approaches to local health promotion, not just for HIV/AIDS.

The case study from Wales differs from the others in that it reports specifically on a health promotion initiative, the Welsh AIDS Campaign.

The main thrust of the campaign is health education, aimed at influencing behaviour, providing guidance and allaying anxiety. This is enacted on an all-Wales basis through the media and by working with statutory organisations. The campaign provides support to individual district initiatives by direct contact with health education officers. The campaign is also concerned with responding to requests for support for training and working with the districts and also directly with the voluntary sector.

A common theme which emerges is that HIV/AIDS has created a demand for in-service and continuing education and has revealed inadequacies in the provision of educational opportunities. This area of health education overlaps with the activity of care provision in that some of those trained will be directly involved in caring for people with AIDS. Others need training because of the nature of their work and the possibility that it may bring them into contact with people with HIV infection or AIDS. In the first group are doctors, nurses, social workers, home-helps, ambulance drivers and a range of other health care workers, including volunteers and family carers. The latter group includes, for example, teachers, the fire service, police, undertakers and refuse collectors.

For most workers this is an issue which will not have been part of their original training, whatever that might have been. The early reactions from these workers were of fear for their own personal safety. In Paddington, the initial staff training relating to infection control was part of the fire-fighting exercise, as was the need for training of community nurses in Brighton when the first patient with AIDS discharged himself from hospital. Since then, staff training programmes – particularly for health and local authority staff – have been developed in almost every district. It is interesting to note the comment from low-prevalence districts such as North West Hertfordshire that, on the one hand, annual updates are mandatory for all staff, while, on the other, it is difficult to maintain momentum when the practical problems are not encountered on a day-to-day basis. Staff may admit to feeling 'all dressed up with nowhere to go'.

Educational programmes for carers also need to look at the social and care needs of this group of clients/patients. The nature of the caring situation is such that programmes do not have to address any situation which has not previously been encountered – it is the intensity of experience which is new. For example, those working in the field of death and bereavement have not in the past necessarily dealt with similar types of problems with confidentiality or infection control.

A common view of training methods is apparent in the reports. As with educational work in schools, there is no possibility that HIV/AIDS educators can directly take on all the training of the many thousands of health and local authority employees in any one district. Various 'cascade' methods have been used: first identifying and training key people in such a way that they can train others and so on, until an appropriate level of training has been achieved throughout the workforce. The report from Bradford offers a note of caution about this method, in that, when the initially trained key workers are not seen as credible by the others, the cascade may fail. Where there was a very carefully structured cascade in Northern Ireland, the issue was not one of credibility but one of assessing when and how the system could best be introduced and explained to facilitate a trouble-free implementation.

More complex training needs are found among GPs who have to take clinical responsibility for direct patient care. Reference has already been made to the difficulties of incorporating GPs in the planning process. They are a group with varied educational needs whose structure of in-service training or education reflects their independence. Several of the case studies relate efforts to provide further education for them. In Brighton and Bloomsbury, there were a series of talks, but in Bloomsbury these had not been well attended and there were plans for more personal approaches through the work of the Community Care Team. The Home Support Team from Paddington also sees its role as being involved in medical education. The personal view from a London GP points to the preferred way of learning being 'case related' and, in the higher-prevalence districts, this may still be appropriate. In contrast, the GPs in areas of low HIV prevalence have shown their interest in this problem by attending meetings in large numbers. The high response rate from GPs to distance-learning packages concerning HIV and AIDS also reflects the efforts which many are making to prepare themselves for meeting the clinical challenges of the epidemic.

A GP working in Edinburgh writes about the difficulties involved in working with patients who are injecting drug users, whether or not they are HIV-positive. His personal initiative has been to stimulate peer group support, to identify educational needs and to make contacts with the appropriate experts. This doctor and his colleagues are not yet having to deal with the heavy caseload of people dying with AIDS, but they are in a position to anticipate it.

In the medium- or low-prevalence districts, each individual practitioner may be in contact with only one or two people with HIV or AIDS. Learning from individual cases may be too slow or incomplete, and a different approach has been taken in Oxford, and further modified in Northern Ireland.

The established success of the GP health promotion facilitators in Oxford made it an obvious choice to build on this model and appoint a 'facilitator for the prevention and care of HIV infection in general practice'. The facilitator's role is to help the practices find answers to local problems and issues; the remit is essentially educational, and does not involve taking on a direct caring role. The post goes some way towards bridging the gap between the institutional and organisational policies and the effective delivery of personalised primary care.

In Northern Ireland, where there are no such precedents, it has been recognised that the most successful approach to a similar goal might be to remain within the professional networks and employ one or two facilitators with a background in primary care.

Health education also needs to address groups with special needs. The Bradford response to its ethnic minorities has already been noted. The needs of people with mental handicap and prisoners are, in some sense, similar in that, by virtue of their residence in an institution, they are denied freedom of sexual expression. However, their educational needs are perhaps secondary to the educational needs of those who, on behalf of the institution, curtail that freedom. Development of appropriate policy and the training of staff in these institutions have to go hand in hand with education for their clients.

People with HIV and AIDS also have health education needs. This has not been addressed as a separate activity by any of the contributors, perhaps because these needs are met on a one-to-one basis through the various client-centred counselling and support mechanisms. However, it is important that we do not overlook this area of health education, particularly when the messages may need to be different from those applicable to the wider public.

Disease prevention

Reference was made earlier to the terminology of preventive activity. In order to avoid confusion with other aspects of health promotion, it can be redefined as those specific individual and technical measures designed to prevent people being infected when the virus might be present.

We have no technological means of inducing immunity in humans or of destroying the virus once a person has become infected. Therefore, passive primary prevention is limited to measures which prevent the transfer of the virus by cross-contamination of body fluids. One means of achieving this is the use of condoms to prevent sexual transmission of the virus. Several of the case studies mention efforts to promote the acceptability, availability and, in some cases, the free provision of condoms. The potential effectiveness of condoms in preventing transmission of HIV may be gauged by reference to the cohort study of prostitutes in Paddington. Prostitute women reported using condoms with clients but rarely with their regular non-client partners. The only three who were found to be HIV-positive were all thought to have become infected outside their working lives.

Blood-borne transmission of HIV usually results from therapeutic intervention or accidental inoculation with infected blood. In the case of therapeutic intervention, HIV was transmitted by transfusion of infected blood or the use of infected Factor VIII in the treatment of haemophilia. This route of infection should now be virtually eliminated in the UK as blood donors are requested to exclude themselves if they believe they may have been at risk of infection, and, in any event, all blood donations are now screened for HIV. In addition, all Factor-VIII is now heat treated to destroy any virus which might have been present. These measures have been undertaken at the instruction of the Department of Health using centrally allocated funds. As such they feature little in the local responses, save for the comments about the need for alternative open-access testing facilities, and the distortion of funding when much of the 'AIDS money' allocated to a region has been used to purchase Factor VIII for patients from a wider catchment.

The other potential route of blood-borne infection is inoculation with contaminated equipment. This is generally understood to mean injecting drug use, but should also include other situations where infection is possible, such as tattooists and acupuncturists. Local environmental health departments have made strenuous efforts to ensure adequate sterilisation procedures. There is also a situation familiar to health care workers where the inoculation may be accidental and the contamination unknown. Needlestick injuries are common, and there are recorded cases where this has been the route of infection with HIV. Safe practice for the handling and discarding of needles and other sharps and the disposing of waste is promoted as part of staff education programmes.

HIV infection in drug users continues to be a problem. Although desirable, the early elimination of injecting is hardly realistic given the current drug culture. Although it may run counter to the philosophy of some workers in the drugs field, it has been accepted that, at least at present, the risks to the individual of injecting with dirty equipment are greater than the harmful effects of the drug. Government funding was specifically allocated for the establishment and evaluation of needle exchange schemes for drug users, and many of these are now being established using local funds.

There are many different models of needle exchange schemes. In Bradford, the approach has been through local pharmacies in conjunction with waste disposal facilities provided by the local council. The service is described as non-judgemental and anonymous. There is little or no link with the recognised drug services, although users are given information on safer sex, a supply of condoms and details of where to find help. In Bloomsbury, by contrast, the scheme is health service-based and was originally located in a hospital casualty department. It has open access, but is linked with the provision of advice on health and related matters. This does not seem to have inhibited its use.

In Lothian, the non-availability of injecting equipment in the late 1970s and early 1980s possibly led to a drug culture based on sharing. The promotion of needle exchange has also required a fundamental alteration in the group behaviour and values of injecting drug users.

Models of care

Although AIDS is a 'new' disease, there is nothing fundamentally new about caring for people with AIDS; we have met all the problems before. There is no doubt, however, that the arrival of the epidemic of HIV disease in the UK in the 1980s has called for a major reappraisal of existing patterns of care. Many aspects of care which we have previously accepted as routine – for example, the testing of pregnant women's blood without explicit consent – have now been called into question.

The clients

People with AIDS are ordinary people whose disease makes them special – 'special' in that they are often young, previously fit people who have to come to terms with a life-threatening disease. 'Special', too, because of the stereotyping and stigma which so often accompany the diagnosis.

For some who are gay, it may bring prejudice and isolation from family, friends and employers, but it may also bring support from a number of voluntary groups and the wider gay community. The articulate campaigning of these groups has done much to promote the rights of people with AIDS and to provide models of care (e.g. London Lighthouse) for the statutory services to follow and perhaps adopt for conditions other than AIDS.

People with haemophilia are more likely to be seen as 'innocent victims' since they acquired their infection, not as the result of their sexual activity, but as an unwanted side-effect of treatment for an inherited disease. On the other hand, injecting drug users with HIV infection may be condemned as 'no-hopers', and those who have become infected by heterosexual contact may be stereotyped and labelled as promiscuous. It seems that the mode of transmission has had much to do with the way people with AIDS are treated and the development of services for them.

The hospital doctors

From an historical point of view, early reports of AIDS were mostly among gay men in London. They were a group who often found it difficult to communicate with their GPs, finding them sometimes unsympathetic and prejudiced. These men were by and large young and fit, with their most frequent health problems being sexually transmitted disease. Therefore it is not surprising that, when they encountered ill health associated with HIV infection, they turned first to the sources of medical help they knew and trusted: the genito-urinary medicine (GUM) clinics. For the most part, this pattern has been repeated in other parts of the country, with genito-urinary medicine taking the lead in caring for people with HIV infection. At

St Mary's Hospital in Paddington, there has also been a shared interest with the consultants in clinical immunology and infectious diseases.

In-patient care

Consultants in genito-urinary medicine do not always have access to in-patient hospital beds. Thus, as more patients required admission, other groups of consultant medical staff became involved. These were very often consultants in infectious diseases because it was thought initially that these patients should be barrier nursed. In some places, such as Brighton, it was the chest physicians who took an interest because they had expertise in dealing with the atypical pneumonias that presented. People with haemophilia were already under the care of clinical haematologists at regional centres such as Oxford and, when they became ill, they continued to receive care from the doctors who knew them best.

In Edinburgh, the pattern of self-referral was similar, with gay men attending the GUM clinic. There was also a large cohort of injecting drug users who were known to the infectious diseases unit as their habit of sharing injecting equipment had led to an increased incidence of hepatitis B. This group of patients has always found difficulty in relating to statutory health service provision, and they have continued to seek help for HIV disease and drug-related problems through the infectious diseases unit.

Before the infectivity of the virus was fully understood, people with AIDS were usually admitted to isolation wards. As the pressure on beds increased and the lower risk of infection was understood, patients were cared for on ordinary wards. At the time, it was considered most appropriate to nurse these patients on general wards and this policy has been promoted in a number of districts where prevalence of HIV infection is still low. However, in Brighton General, the Middlesex and St Mary's hospitals, there has been a conscious move back towards a dedicated in-patient facility. The pressures of AIDS care on the nursing staff are great, and nurses working in these units develop considerable expertise and derive support from membership of a team. However, as AIDS begins to affect every age group and people with AIDS require services such as surgery, obstetrics and psychiatry, AIDS care will take place in potentially any hospital setting.

Out-patient care

People with HIV/AIDS may attend out-patient clinics according to the nature of their problems (e.g. psychiatry, dermatology) or for continuing care and support. This type of support has usually been given by the speciality of first referral, as in Edinburgh where drug users were seen in the infectious diseases clinic and gay men in the GUM clinic.

There has increasingly developed an identified role for health advisers, counsellors and other providers of psychological support. In one instance, a separate HIV clinic (Wharfside) has been established, based on St Mary's

Hospital in Paddington, but elsewhere the arrangements continue to reflect the interest of local clinicians.

Primary care

The problems confronting GPs in caring for people with HIV and AIDS are well described in the personal viewpoint from Paddington. The origins of these difficulties lie in part with the availability of 'alternative' primary care services from open-access GUM clinics: as we have seen, people with HIV infection have often opted to receive care and support from the hospital through the GUM clinic. The GP has only become involved as the illness has become more advanced, which is a reversal of the usual process of primary health care leading on to secondary referral. As confidence increases among patients about their GPs, and among these doctors about their own abilities to cope, the role of primary care in HIV disease is likely to become established. The practical difficulties described in the Brighton report reflect the problems facing all those attempting to provide care in the community.

Problems in primary care have been particularly identified in relation to drug users. For some young people with chaotic lifestyles, particularly in London, access to conventional primary care services may be impossible. The Central London Action on Street Health (CLASH) and the Health Improvement Team (HIT) in Bloomsbury are examples of more accessible services which provide some primary care. Where drug users are registered with GPs, they can bring problems which, as described in the Lothian report, may impose on their doctors' other patients and on partnership arrangements.

Care in the community

This use of 'community' may be ambiguous in that it can refer either to the location of care, or the locus of responsibility for providing care. The provision of care for people with AIDS outside the hospital setting does not absolve the statutory sector from its responsibility to provide an adequate level of care. The needs of people with AIDS cared for at home are no different from those of other sick people: housing, financial support, friendship, home-helps, shopping, meals on wheels, aids and adaptations, satisfying occupation and entertainment, medication, nursing care, physiotherapy, respite care, etc.

The co-ordination of health and social service provision has sometimes proved difficult. The Bloomsbury Community Care Team and the Paddington Home Support Team are examples of initiatives set up to tackle these problems. Their role is essentially education, and one long-term aim might be the provision of more appropriate, better co-ordinated care for all chronically sick and disabled people in the community. Ideally, if such teams are successful in helping all individuals and agencies to work together, they will no longer be necessary and will be absorbed into existing services. It has been pointed out that there is already at least one high-prevalence district where community services are well provided on a generic basis.

The voluntary sector has also responded to the needs of people with HIV and AIDS. The local helplines have formed buddying (befriending) groups to support people at home. Some volunteers have personal involvement in that they may themselves have been bereaved, but many others have no previous experience of HIV and AIDS. It is interesting to speculate on why such support has been mustered for HIV/AIDS when it had not previously emerged to support other people with similar needs, suffering from other conditions.

Terminal care

The principles of terminal care have been well established by the hospice movement, and there are many local teams of doctors and nurses who care for the dying at home, supported where necessary by admissions to special centres. Many of these workers are supported by grants from cancer charities, and there are examples (not included in these case reports) where people with AIDS have been excluded because they 'do not have cancer'.

The case studies in this book describe a variety of models for the provision of terminal care. In Bloomsbury, the Community Care Team is modelled on and is informed by the work of the terminal care team, but, in Paddington, the Home Support Team has yet to clarify its relationship with other workers in this field. In Belfast, despite the low prevalence, there have already been discussions with the hospice movement who have agreed to care for people with AIDS. In Brighton, a former GP, assisted by the 'Help the Hospices' movement, is working alongside the existing symptom-control team to undertake research into the terminal care needs of people with AIDS. However innovative the model of care in a district, it is hoped that it would build on existing expertise and developed concepts of good practice in terminal care, rather than always trying to reinvent the wheel.

The models of care provision for people with AIDS have developed from the original points of referral. There are difficulties for GPs when they are bypassed by patients using open-access hospital services and finally presenting with advanced disease. There is not one hospital speciality 'responsible' for AIDS care (or for the co-ordination of research efforts). A potential conflict exists between the policy statements of low-prevalence districts aiming to care for people with AIDS on ordinary wards and the practical experiences of those who find the concept of a dedicated unit more effective. Difficulties encountered in providing care outside hospital are not new, but attention has been focused on deficiencies and we must be optimistic about the possibility of improvement.

Research and evaluation

Many of the case studies refer to local research projects and evaluation of the initiatives described. At a national level, voluntary confidential reports of people with HIV and AIDS are contributing to our knowledge of the epidemiology of HIV-related disease. In the high-prevalence areas, more detailed studies provide information linking behaviour and risk. A number of clinical research projects have been established to monitor markers of the disease process and to undertake trials of possible therapeutic agents such as Zidovudine.

In all areas, there is a need to establish evaluative research; to identify the needs for health promotion and care provision; and, thereafter, to determine the value and effectiveness of the initiatives designed to meet those needs. New ideas may require new approaches to evaluation and it is important that these innovations are recorded and shared. This book provides one such vehicle for the dissemination of ideas.

Conclusions: The way forward

A review of these case studies, in the context of a model of public health, leads to the conclusion that there are two main types of response, which may even co-exist in one district:

(1) *Metropolitan hospital-based.* Characteristically this type of response is professionally dominated with an emphasis on disease prevention through control of infection and laboratory measures such as screening blood for transfusion. The treatment model is based on open-access GUM clinics with in-patient care in specialist units. This model is most often found in high-prevalence districts.

(2) *Community-based.* This type of response is characterised by multi-sectoral networks involving or even led by the voluntary sector. The emphasis is on health education. Care is provided where possible in community settings with the emphasis on support groups.

The advantage of the hospital-based model was the establishment of medico-professional leadership which set patterns and standards for diagnosis, treatment and care. It also laid the foundation for programmes of clinical research. Disadvantages emerging from this model are that it is centred on the episodic care of individual patients in hospital, and, as a consequence, there has been a failure to develop a community perspective in a planned, organised and co-ordinated way.

The community-based approach places strong emphasis on co-ordinated planning and management. Existing social organisation may need to be strengthened so that the needs of the community can be identified and responded to.

Almost all the case studies in this book demonstrate elements of both of these types of response. The way forward requires the development of community-based responses. The most recent guidance from the Department of Health (DoH, 1989) supports this with instructions to establish co-ordinated local community-based initiatives in health education and to develop appropriate community health services. In the future, there should be no need to replicate the 'hospital-based' type of response, but planners should be prepared to learn and apply the lessons which have emerged. These lessons will not only apply to HIV/AIDS, but may have far-reaching implications and cause us to examine other aspects of health promotion and care provision which we may, up to now, have taken for granted.

The case studies in this book are not presented as models for the future. They identify the questions which districts need to ask about the present state of their services as the first step towards rational and effective planning for future needs in relation to the HIV epidemic.

(1) What is the local prevalence of HIV infection and AIDS?
(2) What are the existing organisational networks? How can they be improved and used to advantage? Who is responsible for planning?
(3) Is there an agreed local strategy with clear objectives supported by comprehensive and agreed policy statements? Do these statements cover health education, health protection and prevention as well as the care of infected people?
(4) What are the arrangements for involving the community in AIDS health promotion?
(5) Are disease prevention policies supported by adequate training in the health and social services?
(6) What are the policy guidelines concerning the medical care of people who are HIV-positive? Are present arrangements and resources appropriate and will they meet the projected demands as the epidemic advances? What are the links between primary and secondary care?
(7) What are the support networks in the community for people with HIV and AIDS?
(8) What evaluation is proposed of present services and how will the results influence future plans?

The case study reports in this book, while they may show many features in common, demonstrate that there is no uniform response to the HIV epidemic, and neither should there be. The only justification for structures and organisations is to ensure that they meet the needs of different localities and different individuals.

References

DoH. (1989) *HIV and AIDS: Resource allocations 1989/90.* EL(89)P/36.

DHSS. (1988) *Public Health in England: The report of the Committee of Inquiry into the future development of the Public Health Function* (Acheson Report). London, HMSO.

Ferlie, E. and Pettigrew, A. (1988) AIDS: responding to rapid change. *Health Service Journal*, 1 December, 1422–4.

Green, L. W. and Raeburn, J. M. (1988) Health promotion: what is it? what will it become? *Health Promotion*, 3, 151–9.

Tannahill, A. (1985a) What is health promotion? *Health Education Journal*, 44, 167–8.

Tannahill, A. (1985b) Reclassifying prevention. *Public Health*, 99, 364–6.

Tannahill, A. (1988) Health promotion and public health: a model in action. *Community Medicine*, 10, 48–51.

Index